SURVIVING AIDS AND CANCER

SURVIVING AIDS AND CANCER

◆

A Guide to Staying Healthy

A Survivor's Point of View

Noreen Martin

iUniverse, Inc.

New York Lincoln Shanghai

SURVIVING AIDS AND CANCER
A Guide to Staying Healthy

Copyright © 2007 by Noreen Martin

iUniverse books may be ordered through booksellers or by contacting:

iUniverse
2021 Pine Lake Road, Suite 100
Lincoln, NE 68512
www.iuniverse.com
1-800-Authors (1-800-288-4677)

ISBN-13: 978-0-595-43152-6 (pbk)
ISBN-13: 978-0-595-87496-5 (ebk)
ISBN-10: 0-595-43152-6 (pbk)
ISBN-10: 0-595-87496-7 (ebk)

Printed in the United States of America

Contents

PREFACE

This book is about my personal journey with two, major, life-threatening diseases, AIDS and cancer. I developed cancer as a young adult and managed to restore my health. This experience taught me hope, belief and to rely upon my inner strength. Although, I did not always go the mainstream route and at times did use some unconventional methods, I found that by having an open mind and a willingness to try new things was part of the key to my success.

Much later in life, I was diagnosed with full, blown AIDS and nearly died. There again, I did my research and developed a treatment plan, which was not always on track with the conventional thinking of the times. Nevertheless, I am proud to say that I do not take the AIDS drugs and I am extremely healthy.

I believe that a great part of my success of rebuilding my health is due to the fact that I do not believe that diseases are incurable. I believe in the old adage "that where there is life there is hope." One of my favorite books in my library is a very old book entitled, "The Book of Health," which has this inscription on the front cover: "You can do nothing to bring the dead to life; but you can do much to save the living from death." This explains quite well my philosophy of health. I hope that my story may be an inspiration to you and will instill to you that incurable diseases are indeed survivable.

1

MY EXPERIENCE WITH CANCER

In my early twenties and after having been married for only a few years, I was working hard and had put off put off having my annual Pap smear for two months. Every visit to the gynecologist, I would complain of intermittent bleeding, which I had since the insertion of an intrauterine device. My previous smears always had shown erosion of the cervix.

Normally, I would experience cramping during menstrual periods, especially on the left side. In the past, my Pap results showed some abnormalities but nothing serious. However, this time was different, my Pap smear came back highly abnormal, Stage IB cancer. So I went from going to work one day at the airbase in Ohio to being an inpatient in the military hospital the next day. The one-day hospital stay consisted of a repeat Pap smear and a biopsy of tissue. The following day I was on an air-vac, military, medical airplane with other patients, being transferred to San Antonio, Texas for treatment at Wilford Hall Medical Center. I had spent six weeks of basic training in San Antonio years prior to this. However, now the circumstances of being there were quite different.

The shock that I had cancer had not fully sunk in. This too would change when a new set of doctors was poking and probing me with more tests and biopsies. The second biopsy wasn't great as I was bleeding too much and had to have the area repacked with special gauze to alleviate the bleeding. By now, I didn't particularly want any more exams, smears or biopsies.

My cancer doctors were quite nice. One was in his early thirties, Dr. Murray and the other, Dr. Massey, a little older and a fatherly type. When the pathologist at the hospital read the biopsy reports, he stated that it didn't look good. In other words, they thought the cancer had spread to other areas beyond the initial site so my doctors informed me that I had to undergo an exploratory surgery so they could biopsy six lymph nodes in my abdomen and leg area. This certainly was a shock, as I had never had as much as a broken bone or any surgery up to this point in life.

The concept of cancer has many stages, the first being denial. It was somewhat hard to believe that I had cancer because I wasn't sick or in pain when I was diagnosed. By things moving as fast as they did, I didn't have time to go through the denial stage. That was a good thing. Another stage to recovery is getting angry. I never got angry per se about why I got this but it has been proven that those who become "fighters" are the ones who will beat this disease. So from that standpoint, I was a fighter. For about a year I would wake up every day and wonder if I my cancer would come back. Having cancer permeates your life and thought processes, especially in the time period that I had it because back then cancer wasn't as prevalent as today and if one had cancer, it was assumed that you were going to die. At that time, having cancer was the worse thing to be diagnosed with; as AIDS had not made it on the scene. One day I decided that I wasn't going to worry about cancer anymore, that I wasn't going to look back and only look to the future. It worked, from that point on; I never again worried about cancer.

Returning to my hospital stay in Texas, I was scared as anyone would be having the prospect of surgery before me and having too emotionally deal with a cancer diagnosis. I always had great faith so I prayed about it all and pressed on. I remember being in the operating room with intravenous drip in my arm with all the operating staff in full gowns and masks. I had just been given a sedative to relax me, I asked, where is Dr. Massey? He came over and held my hand. I told him not to worry as I had prayed about it all and that he would not find any more cancer. Sure enough, when the tissues were sent down to the pathologist for review, the nodes were negative for tumor. At that point, I was stitched up and sent to a room to recover from surgery.

The anesthetic and other medicines did not agree with me, as I became very sick and vomited for hours. Nevertheless, from that time on marked a great relationship with my head doctors and all the young residents. Every day a group of residents in training made the rounds and visited the patients on the ward. Several times a week, we were examined, probed and blood was routinely drawn in the wee hours of the morning.

The cancer diagnosis was starting to sink in and I was given a choice of having total hysterectomy or radiation treatments. I didn't relish the thought of such a massive operation, so I opted for the radiation treatment. Later on, I would have second thoughts about this decision.

After I recovered from my surgery, I started the radiation treatments. For those not familiar with this, it is a simple procedure. They outline the area to be treated with a red dye and the patient lies on the metal table and is given radiation treatments by a very large machine, which rotates around the patient. It doesn't take very long, a few minutes and during the radiation treatment, there is no pain or any sensation. However, there are side effects from these treatments. I didn't have any external burning. However, one of the ladies on the same ward with me undergoing the same treatment, did have some problems. I had 22 of these external, radiation treatments.

One side effect was that I became nauseous after each treatment and the sight of food would make me sick. I was given anti-nausea medication and I found out by accident that taking an Alka-Seltzer before the treatment and before eating did seem to help tremendously. During the treatments, I lost weight. I experienced frequent urination, which turned out to be the worst, long-lasting side effect. Unbeknown to me, my bladder was shrinking right along with the tumor. For year, I would have to urinate several times an hour. Diarrhea was another side effect along with changes in my blood. My female organs were destroyed by these treatments and I experienced premature menopause, which led to hot flashes and night sweats. This continued on for years.

Next, came two, separate radium implant treatments, which consisted of radium being placed in tandems or metal container, I was placed under general anesthesia again and the tandems were placed in the body. I had to lie on my back for twelve hours each treatment while the radiation took effect. Every four hours I was given a shot of Heparin, blood thinner, in the stomach, which is quite painful. Each time I was placed under anesthesia, I became extremely sick with nausea and throwing up green stuff.

Finally, after all the tests, biopsies, exams and radiation treatments, I was sent back home to Ohio and every three months for the next year, I was flown back to Texas for re-examination by the oncologists.

This ordeal was quite an experience and I met other women going through the same thing. I saw small children on the cancer ward and could only ask, why, why must those so young have to suffer so much? My roommate was married with several children and had stomach cancer. Her entire chest area was cut wide open, several inches deep and the wound had to heal from the inside out. I would cleanse out her wound, as her family could not bear to see or do it. This experience taught me to be thankful for life and it taught me about my inner strength, which I would rely on many times later in life.

2

THE VIRUS THEORY OF CANCER

In the early 1920's Dr. Royal Rife found a human cancer virus using the worlds' most powerful microscope, which contained over 6,000 parts. He cultured the virus on a medium of salt pork and then proceeded to inject several hundred mice with the virus. When the rodents developed cancer, he then used electro-magnetic frequency equipment to kill the virus. The theory behind this is that every microbe and element resonates at a particular frequency and if that frequency is applied to it, the microbe will be destroyed. It is sort of like the opera singer who reaches a high pitch note, the same frequency of a glass and then the glass is shattered.

Dr. Rife's microscope was so powerful that he could actually see organisms changing from one form to another. In other words, a virus would start out as a virus, then change to bacteria and back to a virus. This is what is known as pleomorphism.

Dr. Rife had so much success with curing cancer of rodents that he went on to patients. In 1934, The University of Southern California appointed a special medical committee to study his treatment approach to 16, terminally ill patients. After three months, 14 of the 16 patients were cured.

In November of 1931 Dr. Rife was honored at a dinner entitled, "The End of all Diseases" in Pasadena, California. Dr. Rife continued his work but by 1939 the situation had drastically changed. Dr. Milbank Johnson, who was the president of the Southern California American Medical Association, was poisoned. After this other events occurred, Dr. Morris Fishbein attempted to buy the rights to Dr. Rife's machine, Dr. Rife's laboratory was destroyed, Dr. Nemes, a Rife supporter who used his theories, died in a fire along with his research papers and Burnett Lab, who was validating Rife's work was destroyed.

In the 1940's, Virginia Livingston, whom had worked beside Dr. Rife, publicly acknowledged the first cancer virus. In the 1950's some doctors believed that cancer was caused by organisms in the blood. Many believe that the cancer virus is always there and due to negative influences such as toxins, chemicals, poor blood, poor oxygen levels, etc. causes it to be activated.

Dr. Rife never received the recognition that he deserved in life. In 1971 he died at Grossmont Hospital following a heart attack and a Valium and alcohol overdose. Before he died he stated, "I hope I have helped humanity some. I am just one an ordinary man, doing the best he can. We are all here to do our part. Each has a purpose as he lives it and thinks." Such a gracious and humble man still does have an impact on humanity. For those desiring more information about Dr. Rife's life, read the book entitled, "The Cancer Cure That Worked: 50 Years of Suppression" by Barry Lynes.

We now know that certain viruses have been linked to certain cancers such as, Hepatitis B and Hepatitis C to liver cancer, helicobacter Pylori to stomach cancer, Epstein-Barr Virus to Burketts Lymphoma, Retrovirus (BK & JC) to hairy cell leukemia and many more.

In 1955 Jonas Salk was the founder of the polio vaccine, which was made from the kidneys of Rhesus monkeys. In the 1960's, it was discovered that the vaccines had been contaminated with the SV-40, Simian (monkey) Virus. Instead of stopping the production of this vaccine and announcing this to the public, this information was withheld and the production continued until 1963. Later it was determined that up to 61% of all new cancer cases have SV-40. Millions of American children were given this vaccination. The problem with this and other viruses is that they have the potential to be passed on to others and are implicated in certain cancers. Dr. Robert Garry of Tulane University stated that the HMTV virus, for example, has been linked to breast cancer and is likely a cofactor.

3

FOLLOWING MY CANCER DIAGNOSIS

The years following my cancer diagnosis consisted of numerous health issues to include, frequent urination, hot flashes, intestinal cramping when I ate certain foods, and painful intercourse. Since I had not been able to take the birth control pills, the estrogen, hormone replacement therapy didn't work for me either. This started me on my journey to natural products. In the early 1980's, I couldn't get much support from orthodox medicine for natural product. Things haven't seemed to change much in this regard. In that time period, I did find that the chiropractors seemed to be more opened minded about such products.

I started learning about herbs and natural products, mainly at the library, as computers had not made it onto the scene as yet. I always had a natural attraction to the medical and the natural field of medicine. Over the years, I had collected a nice library of health books on various subjects.

In my early health years, I tried to eat healthier meaning not so much meat, more vegetables and eating less sugar and junk foods. However, I must admit that due to work schedules, I did not always eat a proper diet and ate entirely too much fast foods, fat and sodas. I usually suffered from chronic fatigue, which would last from many weeks at a time. I would go to doctors and my blood tests were fine. At time period, doctors believed it to be mostly in the patient's head. However, they now know and anyone, who has suffered with this, knows otherwise.

My examinations for cancer always came back abnormal due to the cell damage from the radiation treatments, which usually meant more biopsies. Although not normal, my urination problems have gotten somewhat better over the years. Several types of bladder control medications were prescribed but without success. Medical tests have shown that my bladder capacity is smaller than normal. I have a higher risk for new cancers developing due to the radiation treatments but I don't dwell on that fact. I have eliminated cancer from my vocabulary and do not plant those seeds of fear into my mind.

My husband and I divorced and I went to Europe for two years and worked on an Air Force Base. After that I lived on Long Island for three years and worked and attended Cosmetology School. I then moved to Loveland, Ohio. I moved back home to South Carolina and took a job at the naval shipyard mainly working on submarines. I loved this job but after eight years, the shipyard closed and this was a traumatic time for me financially and emotionally. Then I was the Port and Facility Manager with a civilian company at the same shipyard but two years later; it too went out of business. That company had a great concept of taking old, navy destroyers and converting them into electrical, power barges for poor nations. The only problem was that the general manager knew nothing about how to do this and confiscated the company's funds by buying hot tubs and spending company money on strippers.

From that time on, I had temporary jobs. At home, I met a man at a birthday party, Bobby, but he was married and I didn't pay very much attention to him at the time. He later divorced and his mother and a friend of mine got us together on a date and we've been together ever since. When I first met him, he was an aircraft maintenance manager for Northwest Airlines, commuting from Minnesota to Charleston during the week. Before long, he had me flying there to see him. His airline wanted him to go to Thailand for a couple of years but he had just meet me and he wouldn't go. His job was later lost due to a major downsizing. This turned out to be a blessing in disguise as he is now back home and he has started a trucking company that is doing very well. We are now happily married and live a normal life.

He and his father started with one truck, which the family inherited from his ex-brother-in-law. My husband solicited business and started an expedited trucking company. In the early year's mom, dad, Bobby and I would deliver the cargo across the country. It did make for some long hours, riding in a bouncy, noisy box-truck but I enjoyed spending time with Bobby and touring the country. Now the business has grown into numerous trucks, cargo vans and employees and it has allowed us to build our dream home.

4

THE TURBULENT STORM

**The person who says that it cannot be done
should not stand in the way of the one who is doing it.
Old Chinese Proverb**

The year 2002 was a very stressful year for our family. My father had open-heart surgery and heart valve replacements. My father-in-law had an aneurysm in his aorta and had to go to Duke Medical Hospital in North Carolina for this special surgery. At one point, my father and father-in-law were in the same hospital at the same time. Later, my mother had gallbladder surgery and my mother-in-law had to have Electro-shock treatments to her heart and a pacemaker inserted. Our parents had numerous health issues to include hepatitis, pancreatitis attacks, reactions to drugs, diabetes and more.

After the parents' health issues had settled down, my brother was involved in an electrocution accident at work and had to be flown to Augusta, Georgia to the burn center. This facilitated family members taking turns driving and staying in Georgia to be near him. Although, he was in a medically induced coma, we made the trip religiously to be with him. This required us to be dressed in cap, gown, mask, gloves and shoe covers for the visit to prevent infections to my brother. It was disheartening to see a loved one who is unconscious, on a respirator and having so many tubes in his body. Years later, he developed a staph infection and developed seizures related to his accident. For a period of time, it seemed like we were living at the hospitals.

About this time, I first developed symptoms of being hyper and having outbursts. I believed it to be stress from all of our families', health issues. My best friend suggested that I go and see her doctor. I did and was place on Prozac, which did help at the time. Although, I did have to have my primary care doctor at the Veterans Hospital, VA, to lower the dosage and I had to take it at night so not to be so sleepy during the day. Around then, I first noticed that my hair was starting to thin and fall out.

The dust had finally settled down in our personal life. Our families' health issues were under control. In 2003, we had an early spring and by the end of March, I had a beautiful suntan from working outdoors. I loved to work in my flower garden but when I did I noticed that when any mosquitoes bit me that I would develop large welts, which was abnormal for me.

The next health event that I noticed was that when I raked leaves, my lower back would ache. This sent me to my primary care doctor who ordered a x-ray, which led to an MRI of the back. A MRI consists of being placed in a large, tunnel-like machine on one's back. Earphones are given to wear, as the machine is very noisy. The test can take up to 45 minutes depending upon the area of the body being scanned. If one is claustrophobic, a sedative may be given.

The MRI showed numerous problems, including, stenous and a herniated disc. I was placed on numerous pain medications for my back and by now a pinched nerve was causing great pain to both my legs and especially when I walked. I wasn't able to walk around a grocery store without being in great pain.

Finally, I was sent to the Pain Clinic at the VA and was given numerous medications with no relief in sight. They recommended a nerve block, so I agreed. I had what is called fluoroscopy, a nerve block procedure involving a live x-ray, which allows the physician to see what they are doing in the back. The down side to this procedure is the amount of radiation that the patient is exposed too.

Before the procedure, I was placed on an intravenous drip (IV) in the arm and given a sedative to relax me. I recall the needles going into the back to be quite painful. The other alarming thing was before the procedure I spoke with the anesthesiologist but in the operating room, a young resident that I had never met, performed the procedure; not so reassuring to the patient.

After this event, I was very happy, finally some pain relief. My happiness was short lived. The pain returned three weeks later. Since there was a limit to how many procedures could be given in a year, due to the radiation exposure and not having great success the first time, I opted not to have any more procedures and would have to live on the pain medications.

During the Pain Clinic visits, I first started complaining of uncontrolled diarrhea. I was having accidents in the house and in public. The Pain Clinic attributed this to radiation from my previous, cancer treatments years ago. Late springtime, I had difficulty hearing and had fullness in my left ear for one month.

I was placed on the antibiotic Cipro and had a reaction to it; it looked like I had the measles from head to toe. I was then given a different antibiotic. Each day now consisted of pain pills, which I did not approve of but I did not have a choice, as I needed to function in life.

My next health issue was belching and GERD or severe heartburn. My primary care physician had placed me on several, different mediations for this and at one point she stopped the Fossamax, a medication for osteoporosis, thinking that it might be causing the problem.

I began to notice that my memory was beginning to fade. I was having trouble remembering something two weeks ago although I could sharply remember something 20 years ago. I began to become more and more fatigued but did not think too much about this as I had chronic fatigue in the past off and on. My fatigue was noted in my records but no special medical tests were performed.

Months later, my memory was getting worse. It got to the point that I was writing down simple things like three-digit, area codes. I realized that I needed certain items from the store but when it was time to go to the store, I couldn't remember what I needed. This whole ordeal gave me an appreciation of how Alzheimers victims must suffer.

By mid-summer, I had large welts from mosquitoes, leg and back pain issues, GERD, tiredness, diarrhea and memory problems. By early fall, my tiredness really escalated into pure exhaustion. I now had heavy, labored breathing. I went to a doctor's care near our home. They ran blood tests, which showed that I was anemic and they gave me some iron pills.

When after two weeks and I was no better, I returned to the clinic. They performed more lab work which showed that I had really abnormal lab reports and I as told to me an oncologist as soon as possible. I called my primary care doctor at the Veterans Administration Hospital (VA) and told her about this. She stated that she would get me an appointment with the oncologist. In the meantime, I got sicker and went back to the clinic, they ran more tests and I was then diagnosed with Epstein Barr Virus. Weeks later and still not having an oncology appointment at the VA, I called to get an outside appointment. All in all, I had over ten doctor visits.

The oncologist ran more blood tests and he recommended that I have a bone biopsy. Due to the cost of the procedure, I knew that I had to go back to the VA for this, even though they had not addressed my previous complaints. The oncologist called my primary care doctor and impressed upon her the importance of the procedure; shortly thereafter, I had the date for the appointment.

Before I could see the VA oncologist, all hell broke loose. For many weeks I could not get off the couch. I had no energy and could not do anything around the house or cook meals. When I wasn't throwing up, I had uncontrolled diarrhea in the house. I was losing weight and suffered with sheer exhaustion. Every day was a challenge with pain issues, memory problems, difficult breathing and night sweats. When I awoke in the mornings, I would have problems walking straight down the hall in other words; I was bouncing off the walls.

After months of being sick and no relief, one day I was at my lowest point. This day I couldn't get any sicker and I thought that I was going to die, right on the couch. I wasn't scared and found it to be the most peaceful day of my life. This experience taught me to no longer fear death and that it is a natural progression that we all go through. It reminded me of one of the coal miners of the Sago Mine that knew he was going to die and left a note stating that it was peaceful. One cannot fully appreciate this unless one has experienced it. It was miraculous, I survived and now I am extremely well and do not take anti-viral or AIDS medicines or antibiotics.

Due to severe breathing problems and wheezing, my husband rushed me to the emergency room. We spent hours there I was given breathing treatments; x-rays, a CAT scan, IV and more blood tests were performed. They wanted to transfer me to the VA but I refused since I felt that they had not properly addressed my health issues in the past. He released me with the stipulation to see an oncologist as soon as possible, which by now I did have an appointment.

After all of this, my primary care doctor was ordering numerous blood tests and one day I had to go downtown twice in the same day for blood work. She also ran two, blood gas tests in my arteries to rule out a blood clot to the lungs. Once I was so weak, standing in line outside the blood drawing room that I had to sit on the floor waiting to get inside. I had tachycardia and had to have an Electro-cardiogram, EKG.

When I finally saw the VA oncologist, he ordered more blood work and based on these findings he too recommended a bone biopsy. For those not familiar with this, it is a extremely painful procedure. One is placed on a table on one's stomach and given a local shot in the back. The doctor then uses a long, screwdriver-like tool and screws it through the skin into the actual bone. Although, up to this point in life, I had undergone a lot of procedures and treatments, nothing could compare to the pain of this particular procedure. Unless one has a strong pain tolerance, I would not recommend this procedure to anyone without being placed under general anesthesia. However, I do believe that it was tougher on my husband who sat through this, watched and listened to my hollering in pain.

After the first specimen was taken, the oncologist determined that it was not adequate and he wanted to know if I wanted to come back for another specimen. I said no way, to get it over with, so he took a second biopsy. By now, I was losing weight and extremely weak. The oncologist could not get an IV in my arms, so he had to give me one in my right foot, which took a couple of hours to complete.

My husband always made time to accompany me on all my doctor visits. He courageously sat through the biopsies, IV's and other procedures. Although, I had no new cancer, my results were markedly abnormal and showed severe immune depression. My health had deteriorated to the point that I had Thrush, a painful infection in my mouth and was placed on anti-fungal medication, which took a good month to get it under control. On 3 Dec 2003, the oncologist ordered an HIV test and it was positive. I was notified on 18 Dec and told to go home and wait for an appointment with the Infectious Disease Clinic. I did not receive this appointment until eight weeks later to the day.

In fact, I had what is termed full-blown AIDS with CD4's under 200 (mine were 78) and many of the AIDS, defining diseases. This misdiagnosis was an oversight by the oncology department probably due to the fact that there are only around 14,000 new, AIDS cases each year in the United States out of a population of 300,000,000. Having a unifying diagnosis was encouraging, as up to this point no one could explain why I was so sick and dying. The diagnosis in itself did not depress me as I had already survived one incurable disease and I was determined to survive another. I believe that this is why I have done so well because I never accepted this as a death sentence. My previous medical experience had made into a strong person and a survivor.

During the eight weeks of being place on hold I was getting sicker and sicker and could only lie on the couch and watch the lights on the Christmas Tree as it slowly revolved around its base. I decided that I could not lie around and do nothing. I contacted a very special person, Tonya, the owner of a local health store. She referred me to an alternative doctor who ran blood tests, placed me on a few supplements and gave me eight, chelation therapy treatments. Chelation therapy uses different types of chelates and hydrogen peroxide solutions to assist with the patient's health. Hydrogen peroxide treatments aid in the survival of the cells.

My husband, my prince, always drove me to all my chelation treatments. After getting settled in the recliner and the IV installed, he would remove my street shoes and place my slippers on my feet so that I would be more comfortable for the two and one-half to three-hour procedure. On chelation therapy days I always felt better and could at least get up off the couch even though I was still extremely sick. Generally, there are no side effects from this procedure except minor bruising, which can occur at the injection site but is quite common with any IV or blood test.

When one arrives for these treatments, a urine sample is given and one's blood pressure is monitored throughout the procedure. The patient is first placed in a comfortable recliner, an IV is installed into the arm and a pillow is given to the patient to rest one's arm upon. The treatment is given in a large room with others who are having this procedure. One is free to read, watch television or to engage in conversation with others. The IV is placed on a portable stand so one is free to go to the restroom if needed. Chelation therapy is safe and has helped many people with many diseases.

Leading up to the Infectious Disease appointment and when I felt like it, I starting learning about my disease on the Internet. I started to relearn good, old health habits and learn new ones. After much research, I started taking vitamins, supplements and herbs. I made major changes in my diet to include eating less red meat and more chicken and fish. I ate a reduced carb diet with a little rice instead of potatoes. I completely eliminated yeast and bread products from my diet. I gave up drinking soft drinks and I had giving up wine years earlier. Cookies, potato chips and other junk foods were not allowed in the house. We drank only non-chlorine and non-fluoride water. Less chemical products were used on the body and fluoride-free toothpaste was purchased from the health store. We religiously took our supplements and herbs every day. I had my husband install a shower filter that eliminated chlorine from the water and chemical products were not used on the body.

On the morning of my Infectious Disease appointment, I had a MRI of my brain that the oncologist had ordered two months earlier due to my memory problems. When I arrived for the Infectious Disease appointment, my new doctors went upstairs to get the results of my MRI. The results stated that it looked like I had progressive multifocal leukoencephalopathy, PML, or possible encephalitis. My doctor thought that my breathing problems may be due to a pulmonary embolism but thankfully, it was not.

I was placed on three anti-viral drugs along with the antibiotic Dapsone. I continued on my natural products but I never hid this information from my doctors. Unfortunately, the medicines had some of the same side effects that made me sick in the first place, anemia, diarrhea and elevated and abnormal blood work. I now was taking medications that was linked to liver, heart and kidney failure, anemia, disfigurement, neuropathy and more, which are not in the original, AIDS defining diseases but are side effects of the drugs. In the fall of 2006, the Lancet, the Medical Journal of England, found that after over 22,000 patients and over 10 years, the patients on the anti-viral medications did not live any longer than those who did not take them.

This day I was given a spinal tap to rule out meningitis plus a flu and pneumonia shot, which I had a reaction to, caused me pain and cellulitis. I was then placed on a second antibiotic, Keflex, for two weeks.

Three months later, after taking anti-fungal medicine, my yeast infection was gone. Then, I was only taking the anti-virals and one antibiotic. Up to this point I had researched and taken numerous supplements to help get me well. Now, I was as good as new and wanted to come off these strong medications. However, I could not get any support from the doctors, as once one goes on the anti-viral medications, one is to remain on them basically for the rest of one's life. I am grateful for my infectious doctors helping to save my life. However, I believe that the anti-viral medications for AIDS should only be used for short-term and when there are symptoms such as, viruses. They should be used as a crutch to assist with the healing process, to level the playing field so the person may get well. To place anyone on these very strong medicines long-term, is certainly going to cause problems. Currently, the number one killer of AIDS persons is not the 30, AIDS defining diseases but liver failure from the AIDS medications.

I continued on the medications for 15 months and during this time I continued to read and learn. I would be up in the middle of the night on the computer looking up information. I had stacks of paperwork all over the office and went through numerous ink cartridges in the process.

The more I researched AIDS, the more I learned that there was a controversy going on about what actually caused AIDS and about the treatment. After much reading, contemplating and serious soul-searching, I decided that the "Rethinkers" side of AIDS made much more sense to me, so I stopped my medications for six weeks only known to my husband whom did not approve. However, due to great pressure from my doctors and a mate, I reluctantly went back on the medications. I was placed on new medicines and these turned me green and elevated my liver enzymes extremely high. The doctors changed these and now I was on a third set of anti-viral medications plus Dapsone. While being on the medications, my blood and liver enzymes were consistently abnormal.

In the fall of 2004, I was given a second round of flu and pneumonia shots, which I had an immediate reaction too. My arm was red with a knot and extremely painful. I again was placed on Keflex for two weeks. However, this time I suffered with pain in my arm, shoulder and chest for six months. After this incident, I refused all vaccinations.

I continued to read and to weigh all side of the issue and found a wonderful book, What If Everything You Thought You Knew About AIDS Was Wrong by Christine Maggiore. Another eight months passed and after contacting Dr. Kary

Mullis, a Nobel Prize winner and the inventor of the PCR or DNA test that the AIDS doctors use to locate the "**antibody load**," I was convinced that what I was about to do was the right thing to do. He gave me that extra assurance that I so needed. I am forever grateful to him for that. I then proceeded to what I termed drug discontinuation day on 1 Mar 2006.

Since I could never get the mainstream's view to add up, I decided that this was my life and I had to do what I believed to be the right thing to do, regardless of who supported me or not. Two months prior to my stopping of the drugs, I found two environmental doctors of whom I think very highly of and they pre-scribed Low Dose Naltrexone to me. This is a wonderful drug that Dr. Bihari from New York City first used for AIDS patients years ago; it is helping so many with immune deficiency diseases such as, cancers, multiple sclerosis, autism and other diseases.

After stopping my medications for the second time, I did so well without them that my husband, who is from the show me state of Missouri, has changed his viewpoint about the situation. My liver enzymes have since returned too nor-mal and my anemia has ceased.

5

HIV

Most people mistakenly believe that if one is HIV+ that person will automatically acquire AIDS and die; this is not so. People have lived over 20 years with HIV and are fine. Also, many AIDS persons are living normal lives. HIV and AIDS are two, very separate issues. Knowing the difference between the two makes them not so scary. One should realize that AIDS may be acquired with or without HIV. Also, great news, AIDS is survivable!

HIV is only one of over 3,000 retroviruses, which happens to exist in every animal on the planet; cats, dogs, birds and humans have them. We have known about retroviruses for almost 100 years. They are the non-toxic part of the cell. Retroviruses have never been shown to kill cells or cause any disease except under laboratory conditions. Retroviruses are passed from the mother to the offspring and not by sex or mating in animals. If goats, dogs and cows test positive to HIV, then it probably is a natural part of our make-up.

So if one is found to be HIV+, don't panic! HIV has never, I repeat, has never been found in human blood or other fluids of the body, surprising isn't it? So one might ask how can someone test positive for HIV if it is not in the blood? Reason #1. In the laboratory a medium is used to produce a reaction to fragments in the blood not to an actual virus. The actual HIV virus has never been properly purified or isolated. Reason #2. There are 70 conditions that can cause a false positive such as pregnancy, parasites, cancer, and drug abuse, etc. So what are the odds that someone has one of these things, which can produce a false positive, pretty good. Reason #3. Even if the HIV test was 100% accurate, it would only prove that one has a harmless, retrovirus. This is comparable to saying that one has green eyes and now there is a test for green eyes. The person would always test positive because one does have green eyes. It would not mean that person has a sexually transmitted disease or is going to die, how ridiculous.

HIV may not be so important and not so accurate either. However, being labeled HIV+ is dangerous because it causes great mental stress, causes denial of insurance labels one with a sexually transmitted disease, place one's name on a list and in most cases the most toxic drugs ever invented by man will be prescribed. Not forgetting that one is being told that one will probably die from this.

In most cases, the person will be placed on drugs without any symptoms. Neither the manufacturer or the Food and Drug Administration have approved these tests for diagnostic purposes, yet individual's health care is being based on this and other non-approved tests.

One might wonder how did HIV, a harmless retrovirus, get married to AIDS? Well, this is an interesting story in which Hollywood should get involved. In the early 1980's gay men on both sides of the United States were going to the doctor sick, dying and no one knew why. For the next two years this problem was called **GRID**, which stood for Gay Related Immunodeficiency Disease, caused by drug use and lifestyle habits. Some were using amyl nitrates, poppers, for the enhancement of sexual relations. Poppers are extremely toxic to the immune system and can cause lung damage, heart failure, severe skin burns and death.

Then in 1983, Luc Montagnier, a French scientist claimed to have found a new virus in these patients. Nevertheless, he had not found it in their blood. So Montagnier sent samples to an American, Robert Gallo, who worked at the National Institute of Health. Robert Gallo modified the samples and then held a press conference and it was announced to the world that **"he"** had found the "**probable**" cause of AIDS.

Robert Gallo immediately filed a patent for an HIV test even though his work had not been properly, scientifically reviewed. Gallo and Abbot labs were raking in millions. Naturally, the French were offended and they wanted some of the patent rights. Both governments pressed Gallo and Montagnier to work out the patent right details. Nevertheless, a federal, ethics committee convicted Robert Gallo of scientific misconduct. Years later, both men admitted that HIV in itself was not enough to cause harm; other cofactors had to be involved. Where are the studies to determine these other factors?

To further simplify this HIV and AIDS relationship, the following analogy is given; AIDS is like having a party. The invited guests are viruses, sicknesses and diseases. The invitations were sent out in the form of drugs, stress, unhealthy habits and improper food. Now, it's party time. No one knows for sure, which guests will arrive or if HIV+ will make an appearance or not. Either way, the AIDS party goes on with or without HIV+. Since 1984, "The HIV Causes AIDS Train" has been rolling down the track pulling carloads of research scientists, drug companies, physicians, fund raisers, AIDS organizations, movie stars, politicians, governmental agencies plus a caboose full of money. It's almost un-American to speak out against AIDS.

Glaxo-Wellcome's (the ex-Burroughs Wellcome) ticket aboard was with Azidothymidine, AZT, a failed, cancer, chemotherapy drug from the 1960's. This toxic, failed cancer drug was given to the world's sickest and most immune-depressed individuals. Most of those on AZT, over 300,000 Americans died and were placed in the AIDS statistics. If AZT failed as a cancer drug, then why did the FDA approve it for AIDS patients? John Lauritsen, a journalist, wanted to know the same thing. He requested documents under the Freedom of Information Act and discovered that AZT was approved based on short, fraudulent, medical trials. This happened again years later with the deletion of negative information about the AIDS drug Nevaripine, "The Good Doctor", Jonathan Fishbein blew the whistle about these fraudulent, drug trials.

Imagine the following scenario, the drug companies make the drugs, test the drugs and then write the reports for the drugs. There is no independent review from a disinterested party. Maybe it's time that we no longer let the fox guard the hen house.

There is another interesting twist to the story. There are HIV-cases of AIDS, which throws a monkey wrench into this theory. As is the case of most diseases, take strep throat for instance, the same microbe will be found in each and every case of strep or else the person has something else and the problem would be looked for elsewhere. Since the 1984 announcement that HIV is the "**probable**" cause of AIDS, the "**probable**" has been dropped and other areas have not been looked into. If HIV causes AIDS, then it should be scientifically proven and in each and every case of AIDS. To cover this obvious flaw in the theory, in 1992 the term idiopathic CD4+T lymphocytopenia was coined, which is a fancy way of saying AIDS but being HIV negative. It has long been established that certain drugs, given for a certain period of time, can induce low immunity or AIDS. This event has nothing to do with sexual contact. Particular groups of people such as, hemophiliacs or organ transplant patients have low immunity due to the drugs that they are given. As long ago as the 1920's it was known that specific drugs may suppress the immune system. This is not a surprise or a new revelation.

6

IS AIDS A SEXUALLY TRANSMITTED DISEASE

**There are three kinds of lies,
lies, damn lies and statistics.
Mark Twain**

According to the Center for Disease Control, every year in the United States there are millions of new sexually transmitted disease cases or STD's. America has more STD's than all the countries of the civilized world. By age 25 half of all young Americans will contract a STD. The highest age group being in the 15 to 24 years old. Supposedly, having a STD increases one's chances of getting HIV. If HIV were contracted through sex and caused AIDS, then the AIDS statistics should be many thousands or in the millions, it is not. The 15 to 24 years olds should have the highest HIV and AIDS cases; however, they have the lowest HIV and AIDS rates.

Out of the 13 million STD's diagnosed annually in the United States most of these are among the black females. Why doesn't the AIDS statistics reflex this? Remember that there are approximately only 14,000, new AIDS cases each year in the United States. The record-keepers like to connect the HIV statistics to the AIDS, which is inaccurate.

For 2003, the top four STD's in the states were Chlamydia 877,478 cases, gonorrhea 335,104 cases, herpes and trichomoniasis with 203,000 cases and the lowest number of 179,000 cases. All of these cases were in the 15-29 age group. Most of the STD's in the United States occur in the South. However, in 2003 the top 10 ten AIDS states, only three states were from the South.

Comparing the HIV/AIDS statistics for the same year, The highest number of cases for the black females was 5,768 and the age group was 35-44 year olds. However, the black male had 11,639 new, AIDS cases. The above statistics are from the Center of Disease Control.

All, new HIV cases have stabilized to approximately 40,000 cases per year in the United States and actual AIDS cases to approximately 14,000. To place all of this into proper prospective, for every one person who dies from AIDS, five to six people will die from Hepatitis C. In 2004 1,192 people died each day in the Unites States from the effects of cigarettes. In a **two-week** period **over 16,000** died from tobacco, this is certainly more than the entire year of AIDS cases and everyone whom develops AIDS do not die. AIDS is not in the top ten causes of deaths in this country. How can we justify the billions upon billions that are being pumped into AIDS research every year when there are many other diseases, which are taking many more lives and HIV has not been scientifically proven to cause AIDS or anything else. You would think that after 20 years, an epidemiology study would have been performed with our tax dollars.

Dr. Peter Duesberg and Dr. Harvey Bialy stated in "Nature", 375, 1995p. 197, infectious units, after all, are the only clinically relevant criteria for a viral pathogen. An alleged virus, which is **not doing** anything, **cannot cause** anything. Cell-free viral HIV particles have never been visualized in any fresh, donated body fluids. HIV has never been proven to be a sexually, transmitted disease. Dr. Nancy Padian has performed a study with 175 couples, where one partner had HIV and the other did not. After this 10-year study, none of the HIV-persons became HIV+. Add the fact that the true, AIDS cases in the United States are lop-sided in the male population. If AIDS were a true STD, then it should be reflected in the female statistics.

There are some other problems in HIV theory one being in regards to Koch's Postulates, the golden rules of medicine; the following are not be fulfilled:

1. The virus must be found freely in the fluids of the patient, it is not.

2. The virus must be found in 100% of the cases, it is not.

3. The virus must be taken out of the patient, be transferred to an animal species and the animal must get AIDS. For over 20 years these animals have been injected with HIV and have not developed AIDS.

The next issue that needs to be addressed is the subject of what the doctors refer to as a viral load. This sound like a real, live virus in one's blood doesn't it? In fact, there is no such thing as a viral load in reality it is an "**antibody**" load. Check history and you will find that having antibodies to the measles or any other disease is a good thing. However, in this particular case it means that one has an incurable disease and other negative consequences, all ruining one's life solely based on a hypothesis, not scientifically, proven facts.

7

AIDS

**Sit down before fact as a little child,
be prepared to give up every preconceived notion,
follow humbly wherever and to whatever abysses nature leads,
or you shall learn nothing.**
Thomas Henry Huxley

AIDS, at times, can be a very serious and challenging disease. If a person has full-blown AIDS, it means that one usually has many diseases at the same time, pulling one's immunity down. However, one can be classified with AIDS due to a HIV+ test and CD4's less than 200 and may not be sick at all. Confusing, isn't it?

To simplify this, here is the current AIDS definition as it has changed several times: A person must be HIV+ and have a CD4 (T-cell) count below 200 or have any of the following opportunistic infections: pneumoncystis carinnii pneumonia, Kaposi's Sarcoma, HIV wasting syndrome, Non Hodgins lymphoma, cryptococcosis, extrapulmonary, HIV encephalopathy, mycobacterium avium intracellular, candidiasis of the esophagus, trachea, bronchi, or lungs, cryptosporidiosis, chronic intestinal, cytomegalovirus, tuberculosis (outside of the lungs), herpes simplex virus infection, progressive multifocal leukoencephalopathy, primary lymphoma of the brain, toxoplasmosis of the brain, histoplasmosis, isoporiasis, chronic intestinal, coccidioidomycosis, salmomella septicemia, bacterial infections, recurrent <13 years, lymphoid hyperplasia, <13 years, pulmonary tuberculosis, recurrent bacterial pneumonia (two or more episodes in a year), and invasive cervical cancer.

You may be wondering how can one harmless, retrovirus be responsible for all of these things, we too would like to know the answer to this. It sounds like if an HIV+ person stubs their big toe, it is blamed on AIDS.

When one has full-blown AIDS, it is comparable to being in a swamp in which one is not being bitten by one mosquito but by many. Even though AIDS is a serious condition, one should not be labeled with a sexually transmitted disease or an incurable disease. When one has full-blown AIDS, one is extremely sick and fighting for one's life, however, survival is very possible. There is no new disease, only a new classification of old diseases. Remember that all of the 30 AIDS, defining diseases were on the planet prior to the 1984 HIV theory. For example, in 1980 if one had strep throat, then that person would be treated for strep throat. However, in 1984 and currently, if one has strep throat and HIV+, then at some point one would more than likely be placed on anti-viral medications and told that one has an incurable disease, based on what, a hypothesis.

When someone has full-blown AIDS, this is as serious as a heart attack. However, without any symptoms or sicknesses, labeling someone with AIDS is unjust. It is not justified to label someone with a sexually transmitted disease either. AIDS is based on a natural immunity of the person, which is earned, whether good or bad. Diet, drugs (legal or street), diseases, past medical treatments, stress, health habits, environmental influences are the main factors leading to immunity. AIDS or one's immunity cannot be transmitted to another person anymore than a toothache can be transmitted to another, it is impossible!

So how does one get to full-blown AIDS in life? Looking back, it was easy to see how I got there. I had a lifetime, an, alphabet soup of unhealthy conditions:

A— Allergies, adenopathy, anemia, numerous antibiotics, abnormal blood work

B— Biopsies, blackouts, bladder shrinkage, breathing problems, bronchitis

C— Cancer, candidiasis, chronic fatigue, coxsakie virus, cystitis, cytomegalo virus

D— Dementia, dermatitis, depression, diarrhea, drinking distilled water

E— Eating SAD (standard American diet), ear infections, encephalitis, Epstein Barr Virus, electric blanket

F— Ferritin (high), fluoride, fractures, fluoroscopy

G— GERD, unsteady gait

H— Hepatitis, herpes simplex, herniated disc, hair loss, hypoglycemia

I— Impure air quality

J— Jaundice

K— Kidney stones

L— Low CD4's, low platelets, lack of exercise and sunshine(low Vitamin D)

M— Mononucleosis, eating microwaved food

N— Nausea, night sweats, no hormones, no supplements

O—   Osteoporosis, over-the-counter drugs

P—   Pancytompenia, pinched nerves, premature menopause, prescription drugs

Q—   Quicksilver (mercury amalgams)

R—   Radiation treatments, reactions to various drugs

S—   Sinusitis, scoliosis, stress, strep throat, swine flu shot, spinal tap, shift work

T—   Tachycardia, thimerosal from vaccines, thrush, toxemia, tinnitis

U—   Vomiting, urinary problems

V—   Vertigo, vaccination reactions

W—   Wrong food-combining, more than 2 glasses of wine at times

X—   X-rays, fluoroscopy, IVP's, cat scans

Z—   Zymosis

The following is a partial list of some of the drugs that I was prescribed prior to my AIDS diagnosis:

Promethazine
Rabeprazole
Fluoxetine
Metoclopramide
Salsalate
Meclizine
Ranitidine
Tolterodine Tartrate
Venlafaxine
Ibuprofen
Acetaminophen
Tramadol
Diclofenac Aldendronate
Oxybutynin Chloride
Lorazepam
Bisacodyl
Magnesium Citrate
Rabeprazole
Hydrocodone 5/Acetaminophen
Nystatin

Amitriptyline
Etodolac
Calcium carbonate
Estradiol crème
Cephalexin
Cipro
Amoxicillin
Sertraline

The above, over time, placed great stresses upon my body. After seeing the above list, you may be wondering, how in the world did I survive that? That's easy, by taking medications only when absolutely necessary and by making the proper life-style changes. More and more positive changes were incorporated and negative influences were eliminated.

I began to re-read health books and completed a Nutritional Course under a Naturopathic Physician. I enrolled in a Master Herbalist Course leading into Naturopathy. I started rebuild my health by taking numerous vitamins, supplements and herbs. Unnatural products were eliminated from my life. I believed in complimentary and alternative medicine. I took the best that both had to offer.

I tried my natural products first before resulting to medicines. If a problem arose, I evaluated my life-style to see what I was doing wrong, what rules of nature were being broken? Health is based on a cause and effect. Positive changes took time as my health was not destroyed in a day, neither could it be rebuilt in a day. The key is to take one day at a time and to stick with it; keep on keeping on as the saying goes.

8

THEORIES ABOUT THE CAUSE OF AIDS

During my initial research into what causes AIDS, I discovered that there are many theories circulating out there besides HIV causing AIDS such as, HHV6A, mycopolasmas, biological warfare, parasitic fluke, benzene poisoning, contaminated Hepatitis B Vaccinations and drug and life-style issues. After investigating these theories, each and every one of them had their own merit.

In 1986, HHV6 was discovered at the National Institute of Health Cancer Center. The virus can infect white blood cells, destroy t-cells and disrupt the immune system. There are two types of HHV6, A and B. 95% of the population has been exposed to the B variant by the age of one. The remaining 5% of the population have the A strain, which is the most destructive type and effects 70% of all AIDS persons. It can damage the central nervous system, cardiac system and cerebral systems.

HHV6A is also frequently seen in chronic fatigue syndrome. It was found that 77% of chronic fatigue syndrome patients test positive for active infection. The parallels of chronic fatigue and AIDS are amazing, as the symptoms are almost a mirror image of each other. As a past suffer of chronic fatigue, I can appreciate the highs and the lows, which this condition can bring.

One theory is that HIV and HHV6 unite to destroy the t-cells. In its own right, HHV6 is certainly more destructive to the immune system of AIDS patients. It is believed that HHV6 mostly stays dormant until something reactivates it and then it causes great damage to the body.

The Herpes Virus Group has several family members to include, herpes simplex, chickenpox and shingles, cytomegalovirus, mononucleosis, herpes virus 6, and the Epstein-Barr Virus. The re-activation of any of the above can cause encephalitis. Personally, I have experienced 7 out of the 8 conditions. I believe that the Herpes Family of viruses is something to take seriously.

A blood test cannot determine the HHV6A virus and a tissue biopsy is necessary to determine this. For now, I have not opted to go that route. However, with all of my past medical issues, I am going on the assumption that more than likely I have the A variant.

Charles Ortleb found that HHV6A infection causes the loss of the natural killer cell formation in AIDS and chronic fatigue syndrome. He authored a book about HHV6, AIDS and chronic fatigue syndrome entitled, "The Closing Argument." Doctors' Knox and Carrigan are doing research about HHV6A. The book, "The Virus Within" is about the research of these doctors.

The next contributing factor to AIDS is mycoplamas, a type of bacteria, which was originally discovered in 1898 in cattle. In 1939 Doctors Swift and Brown connected them to rheumatoid arthritis, in the 1970's they were found in autoimmune disease and later in the Gulf War Veterans. Mycoplasmas deplete the nutrients of the host thus weakening the immune system. There are over 100 known species on the planet.

Being stealth, they can hide in many parts of the body. They have been linked to many diseases, such as Alzheimer's, ALD, AIDS, asthma, chronic fatigue syndrome, certain cancers, Crohn's disease, fibromyalgia, lupus, multiple sclerosis, rheumatoid arthritis and more. Mycoplamas cause inflammation and diseases within the body.

A patent was given by the United States Patent Office for mycoplasma pentrans, which has emerged as a potential co-factor in AIDS progression. Although the Center for Disease Control says that this is hypothetical, some laboratory studies have implicated m. fermentas as a cause of systemic infections and organ failure in AIDS patients. Interestingly enough, special mycoplasmas have been deposited in Maryland at the depository for biological warfare, which brings up the next subject.

In 1969 Dr. D. M. MacArthur stated to a Congressional Subcommittee, "Within the next 5 to 10 years it would probably be possible to make a new infective micro-organism, which could differ in certain important agents from any known disease causing organisms. Most important of these is that it might be refractory to the immunological and therapeutic processes upon which we depend to maintain our relative freedom from infectious disease." In 1969 the Department of Defense, DOD, requested and was granted money to produce organisms to destroy the immune system.

In 1972 writing in volume 147, "Bulletin of the World Health Organization" it stated that they wanted to create a virus that could destroy t-cells. We would test these agents that we make by putting them in our vaccines and see what kind of effects they have. Could the smallpox vaccination been a part of this project in Africa?

Also, in the 1970's experiments were supposedly done taking viruses from animals and placing them in humans. Two such viruses, Bovine-Leukemia and Visna, when combined could effect t-cells. For 20 years it was legal for the DOD to test chemical and biological agents on civilians without their knowledge. After the medical problems with the Gulf War Veterans, this was repealed on 18 November 1997. Currently, Dr. Boyd E. Graves is suing the government in regards to a secret virus program. He has obtained a flowchart from 1971 entitled, "Special Cancer Virus Program." He contends that this is the cause of AIDS.

Another theory to what causes AIDS is by Hulda Clark, N.D. She believes that cancers and AIDS are caused by a parasite, the Fasciolopsis buski, flatworm parasite. She claims that when the parasite is killed the cancer is too. In the case of AIDS, she believes that the parasite establishes itself in the thymus gland causing havoc with the t-cells and immunity. Her treatment plan consists of herbal de-worm procedures and a type of bio-electric medicine know as a "zapper." Although, her theories have yet to be scientifically proven, there is evidence of the parasite, which has been around for hundreds of years and if one believes in the theory of bioelectric medicine, then in theory, this could kill this worm.

The next theory that I discovered that could play a part in AIDS is benzene. Benzene is a hydrocarbon that is produced by burning of natural products and it is found in coal and petroleum products. Exposure to it can cause leukemia and AIDS. Benzene can affect the bone marrow, causes anemia and reduces the immunity, causes fatigue, wasting, night sweats, memory loss, lowers t-cells, cough, intestinal disorders and more. This poisoning enters through the skin and the respiratory system. It is important for those who believe that they have been exposed to it to be tested.

Another theory that I discovered is about the potentially, contaminated Hepatitis B Vaccinations. In 1987-1988, white, gay men were given Hepatitis B vaccinations in California and New York. The vaccine was made from the blood of human donors and later some of these men developed AIDS. In 1983, Dr. John Finkbeiner, writing in "Medical World News" warned that the Hepatitis B vaccine, "Might be contaminated with a pathogen responsible for the acquired immune deficiency syndrome (AIDS) epidemic."

Dr. Alan Cantwell, author of "AIDS, the Mystery and the Solution" stated that, "The CDC, reporting on the first 26 cases of AIDS in the United States declared that 20 were from New York and six were from San Francisco and Los

Angeles. These were the cities that carried out the most extensive gay, Hepatitis B Vaccination trials. All of the first 26 AIDS cases matched the profile of the volunteers in these same vaccine trials, male, gay, under 40, well-educated and mostly white.

The last theory to what causes AIDS is that it is due to the patient's drug, health habits, life-style, and environmental and medical issues. The effects of drugs on the human body is well known, as is the effects of mal-nutrition, stress, lack of exercise, improper thoughts, etc.

After discovering all of the above theories, I realized that AIDS is not so cut and dry and one shoe does not fit all. I decided that I believed that mainly AIDS is due to health habits, environmental issues, medical problems, etc. I came to the conclusion that AIDS is probably not caused by one factor but by many. The more negative influences that are involved in a person's life, the better the chances are for a total breakdown of the immune system. To restore my health, I systematically eliminated negative influences from my life and replaced them with positive ones. Generally, the destruction of the immune system takes time by the same token, it will take some time to restore health depending on how bad the situation is and how much effort is exerted to accomplishing this.

For those who wish to learn more about AIDS Rethinkers, I suggest the following websites: Alberta Reapprasing AIDS Society, Hank's You Bet Your Life, AIDS WIKI, New AIDS Review, Living Without HIV Drugs, HIV Voice, Help for HIV, Alive & Well AIDS Alternative, Dr. Peter Duesburg, Virus Myth, The Perth Group and Rethinking Aids.

9

THE RECOVERY

God gives the mango
The farmer plants the seed,
God cures the patient
The doctor takes the fees.
Old Hindu Proverb

After my health reached rock bottom, I started to re-read old health books and learn new, health information. As I believe that anyone would do who had a serious disease, I began to learn about my problem. I spent many hours on the Internet and discovered that AIDS persons were practically deficient in everything. The more that I learned, the more trips that I made to the health stores, which it all paid off.

After being on various medications and after taking my supplements and eating healthy, three months later I was as good as new. I was a new person who felt and looked a whole lot better. Up to this point, I was taking just slightly over 50 supplements a day, which might seem excessive to most but I was so run down and deficient in everything needed by my body. The re-building of my health made the discontinuation of the anti-viral medications an easier thing to do. Now, I only take a few supplements each day for preventive measures and one drug, Low Dose Naltrexone.

The following are the products that I took to get well. I am living proof that nothing is impossible and that one can rebuild one's health if one takes the time and uses the proper ingredients. In a few cases, I list products by the brand name because I feel that the product is worthy of recommendation. I want everyone to know that I do not sell and do not receive any compensation for the endorsement of any product.

COLLOIDAL SILVER

The healing properties of silver have been known for centuries dating back to the Romans and to the Greeks. In fact the National Space Administration uses silver to purify water in space. Silver is an antiseptic, anti-microbial, anti-bacterial and anti-viral. At the turn of the century and up to around World War II, it was used frequently until antibiotics became prominent on the scene. Colloidal silver is harmless, non-toxic and has germicidal properties.

Colloidal silver has shown to be effective against 650 different pathogens. Unlike antibiotics, germs cannot become resistant to it. The Environmental Protection Agency has stated that an adult could take up to seven teaspoons daily of 10ppm silver for 70 years, without it causing harm.

In the 1990's Dr. Margraf helped to bring back the use of Electro-colloidal silver for treating burns. Dr. Margraf found it to be a wonderful germ fighter. Dr. Henry Crooks stated that in laboratory tests, all pathogens were killed within six minutes as long as the concentration didn't exceed 25 ppm. For those desiring a more natural and safe germ-fighter, colloidal silver may be the way to go. It can be taken internally and applied to the skin.

ALOE VERA

Mankind has used Aloe vera for thousands of years. Aloe has long been used for wounds and burns, to relieve itching, pain and it is a mild anesthetic. I found it growing quite frequently when I lived in Texas. I always had an aloe vera plant in the kitchen in case of burns. It is found to be effective against frostbite too. Aloe can protect against skin damage from radiation and it is an antioxidant. It can help with digestive problems. The best thing about aloe vera is that it contains nutrients such as vitamins, minerals and enzymes, which help to strengthen the immune system.

Anecdotal evidence shows aloe to be helpful with chronic fatigue. It has helped AIDS persons by enhancing the immune response or slows it down where it is too much. Aloe has been used for cancer, bacteria, viruses, fungi, parasites and other infections. Japanese researchers found that it contained at least three anti-tumor agents, emodin, mannose and lectin.

CAT'S CLAW

Cat's claw is an herb, which comes from the rain forest of Peru. Studies suggest that it is helpful in the treatment of arthritis, chronic fatigue, allergies, diabetes, cancer, and herpes, stomach ailments and it seem to enhance the immune system. It contains six alkaloids, which have been shown to enhance the white cells of the body.

This herb can stop viral infections and fight opportunistic infections in AIDS patients. All of the following are attributed to this herb, adaptogenic, anti-microbial, antioxidant, anti-viral, anti-inflammatory and anti-tumor. It has been found to stop the growth of lymphoma and leukemia cells in vitro. It has also been shown to inhibit the binding of estrogen in human breast cells in vitro. Overall, it is a good tonic for maintaining health.

CAYENNE

Cayenne is a member of the Capsicum family or chili peppers, which was first discovered in South America. It is often used for pain, cardiovascular effects and to prevent ulcers. It has a high source of Vitamin A and beta-carotene, an antioxidant. Its Vitamin A content boosts immunity by contributing to healthy epithelial tissues, which serves as the body's first line of defense.

In March of 2006, United States and Japanese researchers stated that Capsaicin could cause prostrate cancer cells to kill themselves. It is also believed that the capsaicin may offer benefits for those with fibromylagia by means of a cream. Some studies also suggest that chemicals in the herb increase the body's heat production, thus increasing metabolism and aiding dieters.

ELDERBERRY

The elderberry has been used for thousands of years. Hippocrates, the Father of Medicine, called it his "medicine chest." Elderberry is said to clean the digestive system and insures a healthy elimination.

Elderberry is a strong antioxidant, greater than Vitamins A, C or E. This herb frequently is used to prevent colds, the flu and sinusitis. I rely heavily upon this herb during the flu season.

LEMON BALM

Lemon balm has been found to have sedative properties and a positive effect on digestion. It has antioxidants in it and has been shown to help those with attention span and dementia problems. Lemon balm contains eugenol, which calms muscle spasms, numbs tissues and kills bacteria.

MILK THISTLE

Milk thistle was used by physicians over 2,000 years ago to treat liver problems. Milk thistle protects and improves its function and can boost regeneration where damage has been done. The active ingredient in milk thistle is silymarin, which protects against potentially, harmful effects to the liver.

Studies have shown that silymarin, silibinin and other flavonoids may be helpful in treating cirrhosis of the liver and tumors. There is good scientific evidence that milk thistle helps with chronic hepatitis.

NEEM

Neem has successfully been used in Ayurvedic medicine for over 5,000 years. It is believed to help rashes, boils, wounds, leprosy, stomach ulcers, chickenpox, psoriasis, acne, diabetes, arthritis, heart disease, blood disease, periodontal disease and it helps to regulate the immune system.

Neem has been found to help with the Epstein Barr Virus and with candida albicans (yeast) fungus. The polysaccharides and limonoids in the bark, leaves and seeds have been used successfully in Europe and India against cancer. Neem has also been used for birth control.

PAU D' ARCO

Pau D' Arco grows wild in the jungles of South America. It contains naphthaquinones, which are potent anti-fungals. This herb enhances the immune system and stimulates the productions of white blood cells.

This herb has been used as an anti-cancer, anti-bacterial, anti-viral and anti-inflammatory agent. It is also uses to treat diabetes, used as a good, blood purifier and to treat yeast infections. Its anti-fungal qualities can be used to treat athlete's foot or nail infections. While growing in its natural environment, no fungus ever grows on this plant.

TURMERIC

Turmeric or curcumin is another tropical plant, which is cultivated in India. It has the power to block inflammation, stop cancer, kill microbes and improves the heart. It acts as an anti-inflammatory by lowering the histamine levels, is an antioxidant, protects the liver and prevents blood platelets from sticking together.

Preliminary research at the University of Texas has found it to be useful in preventing and blocking the growth of cancers. Researchers at the University of California believe that turmeric may play a role in slowing down nurodegenerative diseases. This may explain the low rate of Alzheimer's disease in India where turmeric is eaten regularly. Alzheimer's disease is linked to a build up of amyloid plaque and turmeric may decrease this plaque.

OLIVE LEAF

Olive leaf has been used for over 3,000 years to manage health. It is an antioxidant, which has been shown to lower blood pressure, reduce cholesterol, improve respiratory response, support the urinary, digestive and the immune system. It also helps to normalize blood sugar. It appears to help heart rhythm and arterial health. Its key ingredient is oleuropein, which is thought to prevent LDL or the bad cholesterol. It appears to be an anti-inflammatory and anti-microbial. Olive leaf has been used for oral herpes and in 2003 the University School of Medicine, New York, investigated it for the use against HIV-1 replication.

SHARK CARTLIDGE

Shark cartilage is an excellent source of calcium, phosphorus, proteins, mucopolysaccharides, chondroitin sulphate and Vitamins A and C. Studies have shown that it helps with joint pain, psoriasis, eczema and acne. It has been used to treat gout, dry sockets, arthritis and to repair joint tissue. An excellent book about shark cartilage is, "Sharks Don't Get Cancer" by Dr. William Lane and Linda Comac.

ANTLER VELVET

Although, most Americans are not familiar with the use of deer antler for health, the actual use of it goes back to over 10,000 years to the Chinese and the Koreans. During the Hun Dynasty, deer antler velvet was used to treat 55 diseases.

Deer antler velvet is a natural anti-inflammatory, which contains prostaglandins, glucosamine and chrondroitin sulphates. It has been shown to assist in pain reduction, stimulates the immune system, reduces side effects of chemotherapy, and improves circulation and oxygen levels and displays anti-tumors and anti-viral properties. It contains anabolic stimulating properties and the Growth Factor Hormone IGF-1 and IGF-2. Research in New Zealand has shown that it improves strength and improves muscle response to tissue that has been damaged. It is claimed to increase neurotransmitters in the brain thus cause enhanced moods. It also improves kidney/liver function, red/white blood production and immunity.

OMEGA 3-6-9

Essential fatty acids (EFA's) are fats that cannot be made in our bodies but are necessary for health. Omega's 3's are mainly found in fish and flaxseed oil with a smaller amount being in nuts and seeds.

Omega 6's are found in many oils such as safflower, corn, etc, in the form of linoleic acid. Gamma linoleic acid, GLA, is found in borage oil and evening primrose oil. GLA is important in controlling pain and mood issues, hormone balance and general immunity.

Omega 9 is known as the oleic acid, not being an essential fatty acid because the body can manufacture it. It is found in olive oil, peanuts and avocados. Omega 9's reduce hardening of the arteries, improve blood sugar, reduce the risk of breast cancer and helps to reduce, blood pressure and the risk of strokes.

All in all, omegas offer numerous health benefits. They can conveniently be taken in a combination capsule of all three in the proper proportion needed by the body.

IP6 and INOSITOL

IP6 occurs naturally in grains and legumes. It has been found to inhibit kidney stones, lower cholesterol and aid in sugar digestion. It is also an antioxidant, which has been shown to improve immunity by boosting the activity of the natural killer cells. IP6 is combined with inositol to form two molecules in the body, which in turn helps with the growth, maturity and replication of the cells. According to Dr. Abul Kalam M. Shamsuddin, "The health effects of this combination are greater than of each form alone ... this addition of IP6 makes it an even better anti-cancer cocktail."

IP-6 plus Inositol have undergone extensive testing and no side effects have been found. It has successfully been used with chemotherapy. There is no known drug interactions and it works best taken on an empty stomach.

COCOCNUT OIL

Coconut oil has gotten a bad rap in previous years despite the fact that Polynesians have lived quite healthy on it. According to Dr. Mercola, in 1981 in the "American Journal of Clinical Nutrition", it found that high saturated fat intake did not have a harmful effect on vascular health. In fact, populations who consume coconut oil have lower rates of heart disease. Studies have shown a closer relationship to the consumption of unsaturated oils.

Coconut oil is an anti-viral, anti-microbial and anti-obesity. It contains 50% Lauric acid, which is formed into monolaurin in the body. Monolaurin is the anti-viral, anti-bacterial and anti-fungal which helps those suffering from viral diseases.

We now know that fatty acids in coconut oil do not contribute to heart disease but in fact, are healthy to consume. For those desiring more information about the health benefits of coconut oil can go to coconutoil.com. Coconut oil can easily be purchased at the grocery or the health food store and can be eaten by itself or used for cooking.

COD LIVER OIL

Cod liver oil contains omega 3 and can help prevent heart disease, cancer, depression, Alzheimer's disease, diabetes and more. Cod liver oil is high in Vitamin D, which can be obtained through sunshine, however, during the winter month's sunshine may be limited.

Cod liver oil contains DHA, EPA, Vitamins A and D. The skin bones, teeth, joints, heart, nervous system and the digestive tract require it to be healthy. Since a good portion of our brains is the fat DHA, it is important to have one's Vitamin D levels tested by a physician.

Carlson's fish oil is of the highest quality. It is tested to be free of mercury, cadmium, lead, PCB's and 28 other contaminants. Some health stores stock it and it can be ordered on line.

ACIDOPHILUS

Acidophilus is the most commonly used probiotic or friendly bacteria, which inhabits the intestines. Metchnikoff discovered that people who ate yogurt, which contained lactobacillus bacteria, lived longer. The Balkans is well known to consume large quantities of yogurt and to live well over 100 years of age.

Up to 70 million Americans suffer with digestive diseases. Processed foods often destroy these healthful organisms making it difficult to maintain them in the body. Additives, high-fat diets, alcohol, birth control pills, stress and antibiotic drugs destroy these good bacteria. The effect of antibiotic drugs may last for weeks and may also lead to yeast infections.

Supplying the body with "friendly" bacteria may help with keeping constipation and diarrhea in tact, counteracting lactose intolerance, reducing gas and bad breath, suppressing yeast infections and intestinal problems, assist with separating amino acids from the bile and assist with the production of niacin, folic acid and pyridoxine.

Acidophilus can be found in yogurt, dairy products, sauerkraut, kimchi and brined pickles. Sourdough products contain lactobacillus. It is easy to incorporate acidophilus in our diets and health stores offer tasty, chewable tablets.

IPRIFLAVONE

Ipriflavone was patented in 1976 as an anabolic. Later it was found to be effective in osteoporosis and cardiovascular disease. It is a manmade form of isoflavones, which are found in soybeans. It is thought that ipriflavone improves bone mass and helps to improve bone mass and calcium retention. It is very safe and has no known side effects.

Ipriflavone is rapidly absorbed in the small intestine, then metabolized in the liver. It has a great ability to inhibit the formation of old bone cells and bone re-absorption while forming new bone cells. By combining it with calcium, load-bearing exercise and a proper diet, all go towards helping to eliminate osteoporosis.

TRANSFACTOR

Transfactor is a blend of bovine colstrum, which greatly improves the immune system. Colstrum is filled with growth factors, proteins and immunoglobulins, which support a healthy immune system. It has been shown to repair immune systems that have gone array.

Bovine colstrum has both immunostimulating and anti-microbial properties. It has been used for those who suffer with chronic crystosporidium parvum diarrhea and for AIDS patients. Colstrum is supplied in powder or tablet form.

DHEA

DHEA is a natural hormone produced by the adrenal glands, the gonads, fatty tissues and the brain. It is a precursor of androstenedione, testosterone and estrogen. As we age, our levels significantly decrease. Years ago while having chronic fatigue, I had my levels tested and the doctor placed me on it. It helped me significantly. In women, DHEA seems to stimulate the sex drive.

Some of the benefits of DHEA are cholesterol decreases, insulin resistance and mood improvement. Some claim that it is a fountain of youth. To ensure the proper dosage for this product, a physician should test the DHEA levels. DHEA is now available without a prescription.

LECITHIN

Lecithin is a natural substance produced in the liver. It contains phosphatidyl choline, phosphatidyl inositol, essential fatty acids and chlorine. Lecithin protects against heart attacks and strokes. Lecithin aids in cell function, fat transport and metabolism. It improves memory and is needed for healthy hair. Lecithin also plays a role in male fertility.

It occurs naturally in egg yolks, soybeans, grains, what germ, fish, yeast and peanuts. It may be purchased in pills, powder or granular form.

GRAPE SEED EXTRACT

Grape seed extract is an antioxidant, which contains OPC's, oligomeric proanthocyanidins, which are known to protect the cells and promote a healthy circulation. Two studies, one at the Laboratory of Molecular Medicine and the Davis Heart and Lung Research Institute showed that grape seed extract had a profound effect on wound healing. In October 2006, the American Association for Cancer Research announced that grape seed extract was shown to halt cell cycle and checked the growth of colorectal tumors in mice.

I have found it to be one of the best curative agents around. When my brother had a really bad staph infection and was allergic to the top antibiotic, I gave him liquid grape seed extract and colloidal silver to drink sprayed silver over the wound and I placed an aromatherapy infuser in his room, which dispensed lemon oil. He covered nicely. Grape seed extract is an anti-allergenic, antihistamine, anti-inflammatory and an antioxidant. The OPC ingredients in it are 50 times stronger than Vitamin E and 20 time stronger than Vitamin C. This particular supplement is a no-brainer.

PYCNOGENOL

Pycnogenol comes from the bark of a pine tree in France. It is a powerful antioxidant, anti-inflammatory, helps with skin collagen and to dilate the blood vessels. It is a bioflavanoid, OPC and a procyanidin.

Pycnogenol has 20 more times the antioxidant power than Vitamin C and 50 times the Vitamin E amount. Pycnogenol can effectively neutralize free radicals, which are implicated in at least 60 diseases. There is good, scientific evidence that it can help with swelling of the legs, varicose veins and changes that occur in the skin.

According to the American Botanical Council, pycnogenol protects against lipid oxidation and inflammatory disorders. Christine Chase, MS, RD, states that chewing pycnogenol chewing gum helps to prevent the formation of plaque in the mouth.

ALPHA LIPOIC ACID

Alpha lipoic acid is an antioxidant, which increases the glutathione production in the body. It is part of the first line of defenses against free radial damage. It may help to lower blood sugar and it is a cofactor for many enzyme complexes. It is the only antioxidant that is soluble in both fat and water; this is important, making it accessible to all parts of the cell.

Alpha lipoic acid is capable of crossing the blood/brain barrier thus it is able to go to where it is needed. It causes increases in glutathione levels and thereby helps to prevent strokes, dementia, and Parkinson's and Alzheimer's disease.

ELLAGIC ACID

Ellagic acid is an antioxidant found mainly in fruits such as raspberries, strawberries, cranberries, pomegranates, walnuts, pecans and other foods. Ellagic acid may be a good for preventing cancer.

Dr. Mixon from the Hollings Cancer Institute in Charleston, S.C. has studied the effects of this acid or over nine years. Using red raspberries, it was found to stop cancer division and normal cell death for breast, pancreas, esophageal, skin, colon and prostrate cancer. Tests also concluded that Ellagic acid prevents the destruction of the P53 gene by cancer cells.

The "American Cancer Society's Guide to Complementary and Alternative Cancer Methods" has recognized Ellagic acid to be a promising supplement because it causes the death of the cancer cell in the lab, without harming healthy cells.

It is simple to get Ellagic acid in the body by eating the foods that contain it. Ellagic acid can also be purchased in pill form.

CHLORELLA

Chlorella is a wonderful supplement made from the algae of the sea. It has a natural amino acid in a bio-chelated form. It is a powerful, detoxification agent for heavy metals and pesticides, which we all have been exposed too. It is effective against mercury, cadmium, lead, DDT and PCB's.

Chlorella is great for the immune system and cleanses the liver and the blood. It contains CGF, Chlorella growth factor, which speeds up the healing process of tissues. Studies are underway to see if it can help to reduce liver damage.

It was found that when cancer patients took Chlorella, it helped to prevent the dropping of their white blood cells due to radiation or chemotherapy treatments. I personally take Sun Chlorella because it is derived from fresh water, single-celled, green algae and is full of vitamins, antioxidants, minerals, and nucleic acids omega fatty acids and the Chlorella growth factor.

Chlorella is a wonderful product, which can help to rid the body of heavy metals and pesticides consumed with food. Taking this supplement is a great way to purify the body.

LYCOPENE

Lycopene is a powerful antioxidant, which is found in red tomatoes and other, red fruits such as, watermelons, pink grapefruit, papaya and rosehips. The lycopene content in tomato paste is more bio-available than eating fresh tomatoes. I often open up a can of tomato paste and eat it straight out of the can.

A 1998 study showed that daily consumption of tomato products greatly reduced the LDL oxidation of the body. This is one of the exceptions to the rule, by eating processed; canned tomato products make lycopene more readily absorbed into the body.

It appears that persons who consume diets rich in tomatoes have lower rates of prostrate, lung and stomach cancers. lycopene is great to help prevent cancer and heart disease.

BETA GLUCANS

Beta glucans are derived from the cell wall of Baker's yeast. Beta glucans have anti-tumor and immune stimulating properties by stimulating the macrophages in the body. Dr. M. L. Patchen from the Institute of Armed Forces Radiobiology stated, "Glucan has been shown to enhance macrophage production dramatically and to increase nonspecific host resistance to a variety of bacterial, fungal and parasitic Infections."

Positive effects have been shown in the areas of severe trauma, radiation exposure and in the enhancement of antibiotics and anti-viral medications. Some believe that it is an anti-aging product.

COENZYME Q10

Coenzyme Q10 is found in all the cells of our bodies. It is necessary for the proper functioning of enzymes and other reactions of the body. Certain drugs and diseases can lower its levels in the body.

Animal studies have shown that it helps the immune system function better. The body also uses COQ10 for cell growth and to protect from any damage that could lead into cancer. It is an important free radical scavenger and antioxidant. Without it, we would die because it is needed to convert food into fuel at the cellular level, thus keeping us alive.

Numerous studies have shown that it is helpful in heart conditions, such as angina, ischemic heart disease, myocardial infarction and congestive heart failure. The older one gets, the less is produced in the body. Supplementing with COQ10 makes good sense to protect one's health.

BEE PRODUCTS

Bee products such as bee pollen, royal jelly and bee propolis are wonderful products in which, the bees have done all the work and have predigested them for us. Bee products contain over 5,000 enzymes and coenzymes, more than any other food on the planet. Enzymes do wonderful things in the body to include healing, helping with digestion and protecting against premature aging.

Bee pollen contains nearly, every known nutrient, trace amounts of minerals, vitamins, high in protein and carbohydrates and it contains all the required amino acids.

Royal jelly is from the beehive and is packed with vitamins, minerals and essential amino acids. It can be used for energy, weight loss and immune enhancement. Bees make propolis from resinous substances, mostly from sap from trees. It has antibiotic properties and contains flavonoids, vitamins and amino acids. Propolis is has been found to be effective against breathing problems, gastro-intestinal issues and blood disorders. Bee products are associated with helping numerous systems of the body to include the immune system, cardiovascular system endocrine and nervous system. Bee products are available in powders, liquids, tablets, pills, and capsules and don't forget honey.

THYMUS SUPPLEMENTS

The thymus gland is located at the top portion of the chest and is an endocrine gland. The thymus produces hormones, which strengthen the immune system. However, by age 25 the thymus shrinks and one is more susceptible to tumors and other serious disorders. To compensate for this, thymus supplements can be taken to ward off infections and strengthen the immune system.

The thymus is responsible for the producing T lymphocytes or the T-cells, which are responsible for "cell-mediated immunity", meaning not controlled by antibodies. During my healing process, I purchased thymus, glandular products from the health store. These products are claimed to help with Hepatitis B and C, rheumatoid arthritis, systemic lupus, multiple sclerosis, psoriasis, certain skin cancers, allergies, herpes and chronic fatigue.

Glandulars, being more popular in Europe, have a long and safe history. They target a specific organ and provide it with the nutrient that it needs.

COLLOIDAL MINERALS

The majority of the human body is comprised of minerals. According to Dr. Gary Price Todd, the body needs 60 minerals to maintain health. Today's soil contains 16 to 20, which means that plants and humans lack the necessary minerals.

In Utah there is a TRC Mine, which mines plant minerals that were covered by a glacier. These particular minerals are water-soluble and are easily digested by the body. The significance of water-soluble minerals is that they are nearly ten times more bio-available at the cellular level than metallic minerals.

These minerals are leached from pre-historic plants in large, food vats and are free of contaminants. These minerals are completely organic and have a negative charge to form a direct hydrogen bond with water providing superior water solubility, which makes for easy digestion. Anyone who takes one ounce of this product daily is supplying the body with 75, plant, derived minerals to help maintain health.

Another great product that this company offers is called Liquid Life Complete. It is an all-in-one nutritional supplement for those on the go who for those who do not wish to swallow a bunch of pills. One ounce of Liquid Life Complete supplies 75, colloidal minerals, 16 vitamins, and antioxidants, 18 amino acids, 15 herbs, aloe vera and other nutrients.

This product is excellent for those desiring to maintain health. Some of the herbs that it contains are green tea extract, ginkgo bilboa, red raspberry leaf, grape seed extract, Pau d'Arco, cat's claw and many more. All in all, there are 128 nutrients at a very affordable price, being in the best form to ingest and be absorbed into the body, as a liquid. I usually mix the product with some type of juice in the mornings. Those desiring more information about this great product should go to www.reachforlife.com

B COMPLEX VITAMINS

The B complex of vitamins is a group of eight vitamins. Vitamin B1 is more commonly called thiamin and comes from rice. B2 is also called riboflavin and aids in metabolizing fats, carbohydrates and proteins. It is also needed to produce red blood cell and for good health. B3 or niacin is a water-soluble vitamin, which is needed for growth and reproduction. B6 or pyridoxcine maintains nerve and muscle cells and works to control the levels of the amino acid homycysteine. B9 is known as folic acid and is needed to synthesize adrerine and thymine, which help to make up our genes, DNA and chromosomes. B9 is also needed for the metabolism of the methionine, an amino acid that is found in animal proteins. B12 or cyanocobalimin is needed to build nerve cells, red blood cells and to make DNA in the cells. It is claimed to help those who are tired and is best taken in a sublingual form where 98% of it can be directly absorbed into the body.

Pantothenic acid is required for growth, reproduction and physiological functions of the body. It is needed to break down carbohydrates, proteins and fats. Biotin is needed for cell growth, the production of fatty acids and to metabolize fats and amino acids. The B complex of vitamins is essential for those who wish to improve, skin, hair and nails.

CALCIUM

Most everyone knows that calcium is needed for strong bones and teeth. However, it is also needed in every cell of the body for muscle functioning, nerve transmissions, blood clotting and more. Calcium is also good for the heart and may lower blood pressure.

Getting enough calcium, Vitamin D, phosphates and magnesium helps to build strong bones. Supplementation with calcium is essential as most people drink fluoridated water and liquids, which displaces the calcium in the body.

MAGNESIUM

Magnesium is the fourth, most abundant mineral in the body with 50% of it being in our bones. Magnesium is required for over 300 biochemical reactions in the body. It helps to maintain muscles and nerves, steadies heart beats, supports the immune system, helps to regulate blood sugar and blood pressure and is involved in energy metabolism and protein synthesis. Therefore, magnesium supplementation should be high on one's list. An easy way to get magnesium into the body is to soak in the tub with good, old-fashioned Epsom Salt.

VITAMIN C

Vitamin C, also known as ascorbic acid, is a water-soluble antioxidant. It helps in the formation of collagen, helps to maintain capillaries, bone and teeth.

It also helps the immune system to fight off intruders and tumor cells. It supports the cardiovascular system and assists with the nervous system.

Dr. Linus Pauling noted that terminally ill, cancer patients lived four times longer than those subjects who did not receive Vitamin C did. Many studies have confirmed Vitamin C to be an effective anti-cancer agent.

VITAMIN E

Vitamin E is a family of eight antioxidants and is fat-soluble. Vitamin E protects Vitamin A, protects essential fatty acids from oxidation and prevents the breakdown of tissue. It is claimed to help prevent cancer, heart disease, cataracts and assist with leg cramps.

Vitamin E is safe in doses up to 1,000mg/day. Researchers found that 800iu per day helped to lower LDL cholesterol.

ZINC

Zinc is a mineral, which is necessary for the immune system, healing of wounds, for growth, digestion and reproduction, to control diabetes and is needed for taste and smell. Zinc is also known for its ability to prevent or ease colds, due to improving the white blood count. Zinc has been used to assist persons with AIDS to increase immunity. Zinc, a wonderful mineral, also helps to absorb minerals and aids in regulating hormones.

SELENIUM

Selenium is a trace element, which plays a role in the antioxidant enzyme glutathione peroxidase, an important factor in helping to ward away free radial damage to the body at the cellular level. Since we live and die at the cellular level, selenium is a necessary element to prevent chronic disease, premature aging, heart attacks and more. Areas with high selenium levels in the soil have been shown to have lower rates of cancer. An easy way to get selenium into the diet is to eat Brazil nuts. Each nut contains approximately 100mg of selenium. At the height of my illness, I was consuming ten Brazil nuts a day or 1,000mg of selenium.

AMINO ACIDS

Amino acids are building blocks, which build proteins and enzymes. They also repair and form antibodies to help fight bacteria and viruses and carry needed oxygen throughout the body. There are 22 amino acids of which nine are essential and cannot be produced by the body. Amino acids can be taken individually or as a group. An excellent source of all 22 amino acids is honey.

DIGESTIVE ENZYMES

Digestive enzymes assist with digestion by breaking down foods and nutrients into forms absorbable by the body. They can help with indigestion, heartburn, cramps and gas. My father-in-law suffers from pancreatitis attack and I recommended that he take them and as long as he stays on them, he doesn't have any attacks.

Enzymes can prevent and neutralize stomach acid and prevent irritable bowel syndrome. These enzymes are available with protease, amylase, lipase, cellulose, pepidase, maltase and lactose. All of the above respectively work to break down proteins, carbohydrates, fat, cellulose, peptides, and malt sugar and milk sugar.

Anti-acids in the long run do more harm than they do good and may mask a symptom that needs to be addressed. Heartburn can indicate, ulcers, cancer or heart problems. When hydrochloric acid is blocked, the digestive process is not complete. Too much hydrochloric acid gives the same symptoms as too little so any unusual symptom needs to be addressed by medical personnel.

It is a fact that enzymes can strengthened the immune system, especially the natural killer cells. Digestive enzymes come in various types and flavors and may be purchased at the health store.

ESSIAC

Essiac or the brand that I take is called "Just Tea". Essaic is named after a nurse named Ciasse spelled backwards. It is an herbal preparation that she was given in the1920's by Indians from Canada to cure cancer. The four herbs in it are Burdock Root, Sheep Sorrel, Slippery Elm Bark and Turkey Rhubarb Root.

These herbs work to neutralize blood toxins, detoxify the liver and inflammations. A healthy liver is extremely important for good health, as the liver has to deal with all of the toxins and medicines that it is exposed too.

OIL OF OREGANO

Oil of oregano is an anti-fungal, which comes from 100% Mediterranean oregano. It has a long list of uses, some being for staph infections, strep throat, e-coli, candidiasis and many more infections. One great product is P73, which contains a high concentration of oregano and oxidants.

NAC

N-acetylcysteine (NAC) is a form of cysteine, an amino acid. It is used for respiratory disorders such as, bronchitis, used to break down mucus, protects the liver, and synthesizes glutathione.

Dr. Robert Clark stated that, "Now that we're identified low glutathione levels in males with brain injuries, we can begin looking at NAC as a life-saving treatment for those injuries." The National Institute of health found that NAC reduces cravings for cocaine.

Some natural means of NAC are found in wheat germ, granola, oat flakes, ricotta, yogurt, sausage, pork, chicken and luncheon meats.

SOD

Superoxide dismutase or SOD is a naturally occurring antioxidant in the body. At birth we are given three antioxidants, SOD, gluthathione peroxidase and catalase. When our SOD levels are hindered, we develop respiratory problems, memory loss, and vision problems, cardiovascular issues and premature aging.

In the past, taking SOD was a problem because the strong gastric juices of the stomach caused it to be destroyed. French scientists discovered that by adding cucumus melo (a melon high in SOD) and a wheat stabilizer, it was then possible to prevent this destruction. This product is called Glisodin.

DMG

Dimethylglycine (DMG) is a non-protein found in plant and animal cells. It is the building block for hormones, neurotransmitters and DNA. It improves the oxygen levels, prevents lactic acid build-up and is stimulates the immune system.

Studies have found it to help compulsive behavior in autistic person. DMG can assist the damaged heart to be able to better utilize oxygen. Having DMG in a first-aid kit is not such a bad idea. The pills are extremely small and can dissolve in the mouth.

NONI

Noni is the juice from the Indian mulberry, which grows in the South Pacific Islands. According to Dr. Ray Sahelian, noni contains anthraquinones, organic acids, xeronine, beta-carotene, niacin, riboflavin, thiamin, minerals, iron, calcium, caprylic acids, Vitamin C and alkaloids.

Noni helps cholesterol levels, reduces triglycerides and the immune system. It has a component called noni-ppt, which is claimed to be anti-tumor. Noni is available in capsule or in liquid form.

IMMUNE 247

This is a product that I took religiously, which contains beta-glucans and other polysaccharides, immune stimulating components coming from mushrooms and a compound from green tea. Each 500mg capsule contains agaricus blazei, sinensis, maitake, shittake, coriolus versicolor, reishi, cordyceps and EGDG from green tea.

Mushrooms have long been used for their immune and medicinal qualities. This product may be used with cancer treatments and surgeries. Studies performed in China and Japan show these mushrooms are anti-cancerous. Today, most of our antibiotics come from fungi. For those desiring to boost their natural killer cells, interferon, interleukin, tumor necrosis factor, t-cells, macrophages and more, this product is highly recommended.

ABM EXTRACT

Another wonderful, mushroom product is ABM Extract or agarictus blazei. It too is full of beta glucans, which are immune stimulating. Japanese studies have shown it to be the have the best, anti-cancer effects of all mushrooms. It has also been shown to be useful for pneumonia in vitro.

REVIVO

Revivo is a brand name for a mix of 12 of the finest, Chinese herbs, which help to activate the immune system to fight viruses. The extracts are in the form of a tea, which is taken daily. It has somewhat of a bitter taste but its flavor can be improved with the addition of a little sugar or honey. I found this tea to be quite pleasant and one of the herbs or a combination of several caused my eyesight to improve so that I did not need my reading glasses while on the product.

Revivo is being used to treat AIDS patients in the Far East. The Revivo website has a wealth of information about the product and some of the results of people who are on it. For more information, go to natureproducts.net/Medcine/Revivo.html.

10

THEORIES OF MEDICINE

**As long as there is breath in my body I will ever be a seeker of the truth.
from the Altered States Website**

Early on my journey to health, I discovered that many years ago there was a difference of opinion into what caused disease. There were two theories of medicine, the germ theory and pleomorphism. The germ theory of medicine is based on monomorphism or one form. This theory goes way back centuries ago to Pliny and was later extended by the botanist Linnaeus. A couple of centuries ago, Pasteur of Paris and Professor Koch of Berlin, also believed the germ theory to be true.

Professor Koch formulated the germ theory laws, Koch's Postulates, which are still used today. They proclaim the following:

1. it must be demonstrated.

2. that it is constantly present in the fluids of tissues of the individual subject to that disease.

3. its absence from all other diseases.

4. its isolation, growth and repeated cultivation on proper culture media.

5. Its power of reproducing the disease after inoculation in susceptible animals.

The germ theory believes that germs are the cause of diseases and when a person is ill, these germs are being thrown off in the waste of the body such as urine, sweat, etc. The germ theory believes that germs should be attacked with medicines. When one is sick or dying, this may be an appropriate approach. However, unless steps are taken to prevent the situation, the problem will occur again and possibly in a worse form.

Ploemorphism means many forms. Its roots go back over 200 years to Almquist, Bergstrand, Enderlein and to Bechamp, an adversary of Pasteur and others. Some modern believers of this theory are Gaston Naessens, the late Royal Rife, Dr. Robert Young and Dr. Dennis Myers.

This theory proposes that germs start out in the body as small forms called microzyma, somatids or protits. These protits change into viruses, bacteria, fungus and back to the original form. Dr. Myers believes that they go through a 16-stage cycle. These change forms produce waste, which causes us pain, sickness and disease.

Disease is our common enemy but nature is our friend if we will obey her laws. With pure blood on our side, we can win the fight. But weakening the body by abusing drugs, alcohol, tobacco, improper food, over-eating, wrong-food combining, lack of exercise and sleep, over-worked and negative thinking, makes the body's soil or PH becomes fertile for the planting of germs or disease.

There is a vast difference in the philosophy between the germ theory and pleomorphism. Therefore, the treatment approach would be different. Interestingly enough, Pasteur, the Father of Modern Medicine, was claimed to have stated on his deathbed that Bechamp was right, the terrain (PH) is everything and the germ is nothing. I decided that pleomorphism makes more sense to me, for example, when two neighbors plant the same flowers, each is exposed to the same sun and rain. Why did one neighbor have a beautiful flower garden and the other did not? Could one of them have used the proper fertilizer to aid the soil and thus produce the beautiful garden? By the same token, how many times have an entire family been exposed to a bug yet not every one in the family gets sick? Could the person's terrain or PH have anything to do with this? I believe that it does.

For those who believe that PH is important to one's health, litmus paper can be purchased at the health stores for testing the PH of urine and saliva. 7.3 is a good PH for saliva and one must remember that one number to the next on the scale jumps ten-fold in the degree of alkalinity, a significant increase. A healthy diet consists of eating 80% alkaline foods to 20% acid-forming foods. The following lists the alkaline and acid-forming foods:

ALKALINE FOODS
(EAT 80%)

ALMONDS	LETTUCE
APPLES	LIMA BEAN

BANANAS

MOLASSES

BEAN (DRIED)

MUSHROOMS

BEETS

ONIONS

BROCCOLI

ORANGES

BRUSSEL SPROUTS

PEACHES

CABBAGE

PEARS

CARROTS

PEAS

CAULIFLOWER

PINEAPPLE

CELERY

POTATOES

CUCUMBERS

RADISHES

DATES

RAISINS

FIGS

SAUERKRAUT

GRAPEFRUIT

SPINACH

GREEN BEANS

STRAWBERRIES

LEMONS

TOMATOES

WATERMELON

ACID FOODS
(EAT 20%)

BACON

LENTILS

BEEF

MILK

BLUEBERRIES

MACRONI

BRAN

OATMEAL

BREAD (WHEAT)

PEANUT BUTTER

BUTTER

PORK

CHICKEN

RICE

COD

SALMON

CORN

SCALLOPS

CRACKERS

CRANBERRIES

PLUMS

EGGS

FLOUR

HONEY

SHRIMP

SQUASH

SUNFLOWER SEEDS

TURKEY

WALNUTS

WHEAT GERM

11

FOOD ELEMENTS AND COMBINING

I discovered to maintain a state of health, it was important to understand what the human body needs to survive. A normal human needs 16 elements to survive. Every time we think, blink, wink, and talk or move, a portion of these elements is consumed. These worn out elements must be replaced to stay alive. Therefore, when we eat, we should keep in mind to replace these consumed elements. Disease and death are largely because we overeat on some of these elements and under-eat on others. Over-weight people are a prime example of this, being overly fed on sugary and starchy foods and underfed on others.

Foods can be divided into 4 classes, proteins, carbohydrates, fats and mineral salts. Proteins are used in the body to build up or repair worn-out tissues. Food rich in proteins are fish, meat, eggs, beans, etc.

Carbohydrates are fuels for the body. They give heat and energy. We ordinarily mean sugar and starch. However, an over supply of starches will be stored up in the body as fat.

Fats are foods, which are usually rich in the elements of carbon, hydrogen and oxygen such, butter, cream, cheese, olive oil, etc.

Mineral salts are found in most foods and should be distinguished from ordinary table salt. They form the cells and are so important, that if one of these mineral salts is removed, the remaining salts fail to function properly. The discovery of vitamins was a wonderful, step-forward, but the discovery of mineral salts is vastly more important because when mineral salts are removed from our food, all the vitamins are automatically removed too.

When one or more of the mineral salts are diminished, sickness and eventually death will follow both in the vegetable and the animal kingdom. For instance, the least amount of iodine removed from our food will affect the thyroid gland and when the iodine disturbance is sufficient, goiter will soon develop.

Mineral salts play an important and indispensable part in the process of elimination. There is not a single organ, tissue, cells in the body that is not absolutely dependent upon mineral salts. They play an important part in metabolism, preserving tissues from putrefaction (rotting), regular chemical reactions of the internal secretions and the blood, assist in iron formation and more.

Dr. Linus Pauling stated that all diseases go back to a mineral deficiency. The important thing to remember is that the slightest amount of mineral salts added or removed from our food is likely to convert the best food into the deadliest of all poisons. Fruits and vegetable are rich in these life-giving mineral salts and it is important to know that cooking dissolves some of them so it is preferable to eat them raw. Nature's finest and the most wholesome sugar is fruit sugar. The fresh juice of sweet grapes, pears, oranges and other sweet fruits are pre-digested and therefore are ready for immediate absorption into the body.

Other fruits such as, apples, grapes, oranges, plums, peaches, pineapples and juicy berries possess great germicidal properties in addition to their food value. The old saying that an apple a day keeps the doctor away has some merit. Fruits as it has been supposed, do not acidify the body, except cranberries do. The organic acid found in fruits and vegetables is not free but combine with bases or alkaline substances. During digestion these salts are decomposed in the fluids of the tissues, the acids are set free and burned as carbon dioxide. The alkaline base that is left enters into combination with the acid wastes and neutralizes the acids in the tissues.

Remember that it is important to steam vegetable so not to destroy the vitamins and mineral salts. I found that rice cookers make excellent steamers for most vegetables. If I cooked vegetables, I saved the water to drink or to be used in soups. I never soaked meat and vegetables in water because this destroys most of the nutrients. I kept the peelings of potatoes, apples, etc. because the mineral salts lie next to the outer covering.

I never microwaved food because research by the Russians has shown that people who eat microwaved foods showed a statistically higher incidence of stomach and intestinal cancer. Also, malfunctions occur within the lymphatic system due to chemical alterations within the food. Microwaves generate a chemical, acrylamide, which causes cancer. Also, like the heating of foods, microwaves decrease the nutritive values of foods and the bioavailability of the vitamins and minerals. Dr. Hans Hertel discovered that people who ate microwaved food had changes in their blood chemistry to include a decrease in hemoglobin and cholesterol values, a weakened immune system and an increase in leukocyte levels, which indicates damage to the cells.

According to Larry Cook, from the "Idaho Observer", a simple test is to take two pots and plant with seeds. Water one pot with microwaved water and the other with tap water. The microwaved plant will not grow. Think about food that is microwaved and the harm that it is doing in the body. I think that I will try this experiment with heated water from the stovetop and see if the plant will grow.

FOOD COMBINING RULES

Most people may be unaware that there are rules for eating or combining foods together. Most people just push anything into their mouth, which winds up in the stomach, not aware that because of this they experience heartburn and other digestive problems. As far back as the 1920's, a holistic doctor by the name of Sheldon, and many others were aware of these rules. Many progressive doctors now also realize the importance of food combining to alleviate digestive problems.

Proper food combining is essential to our health. Starch begins digestion in the mouth and passes through the stomach with little change. Meat or proteins are not digested in the mouth but by the digestive juices of the stomach. Therefore, the less we chew meat, the better. However, the more we chew other foods the better.

Remember that life requires proteins and carbohydrates but not at the same meal. In reality there are hundreds of foods to choose from while observing the following food combining rule, which will make for a healthy digestion:

The fewer kinds of foods one eats at any meal, the better.
Eat only one kind of protein at a meal and eat plenty of green, leafy vegetables.
Never eat 2 kinds of proteins at a meal, ex. meat and eggs.
Never eat starches and proteins at the same meal, ex. bread and meat.
Eat starches like potatoes with green vegetables or salads.
Never eat two starches at the same meal, ex. bread and potatoes.
Never combine fruit with starches.
Eat salads at the start of meals and remember that salads can be freely eaten.
Milk combines nicely with fruits and vegetables but not proteins.
Fruit combines well with vegetables, nuts and dairy products.
Apply the above rules to eating soups.
Get all of the elements in a day's ration but it is not necessary to get them in one meal.

No food is perfect by itself. Most require other foods to be added to balance what they are lacking, for example, milk is almost a perfect food but it can be improved on by the additions of fruit. Green vegetable tops are rich in vitamins and mineral salts but they need proteins and starches to complete them. Protein builds tissues but it needs salads, fruits, vegetables and starches to complete them. Bottom line, food can be improved by the addition of some other, certain food. One note about nuts, they are excellent for health but need to be thoroughly chewed to a liquid to ensure proper digestion.

12

HOW TO LIVE A LONG AND HEALTHY LIFE

Get normal blood and you will have perfect health and long life.
A. B. Shinn

In my quest for health, I realized that in regards to food we lead an artificial existence. We eat denatured, processed and the wrong kinds of foods together. Humans, being intelligent beings, are the only animals on the planet that heats, processes and destroys their food. When we subsist mainly on white bread, peeled potatoes, white sugar, processed foods, sodas, etc., all of which are lacking in the health-giving mineral salts, vitamins, digestive ferments and amino acids, how long can we expect to remain healthy?

If we want to enjoy a long life, we cannot get it from wishing and hoping or from a fountain of youth. Health can only be acquired by the obedience to the laws of nature, by complying with her laws. Around the world there are people who live long lives, such as the Bulgarians. Their climate and rainfall is similar to ours. They live in farm communities and remain healthy by eating fruits, nuts, vegetables and milk. Their food makes their blood almost perfect in repairing the body.

Scientific experiments have concluded that chronic or degenerative diseases can be prevented by the eating of balanced meals and by using correct-eating habits. Nature has so very wisely placed in foods all the elements to keep us healthy. When we eat unbalanced diets and have improper, health habits, our tissues start to slowly weaken and thus prepared the way for germs and disease. The arteries, heart, kidneys, liver and other vital organs become damaged, which produces attacks, chronic problems and premature death.

Every time our blood fails to provide the correct nutrient to the cells, the space is filled with connective tissue, which is tough, cartilaginous tissue. This tissue causes us to become less active because we now have less cell life in the body. By keeping the blood normal and supplied with the correct cell-building food and favorable conditions, can the length of life be lengthened.

If one's blood is 70% normal for hemoglobin, one is 30% below normal in muscle, glands, nerves and brain; that is 30% blank, a failure in thoughts, works and deeds. This markedly, lowered vitality and energy is preventable. Old age is only one aspect of toxemia. When our blood is improperly nourished, it cannot supply the cells with needed material and thus preventing the formation of connective tissue, consequently we become stiff and inactive. Wrong food produces wrong tissue; wrong tissue produces premature aging.

Drugs cannot become a part of the body, only food can become a part of the human body and only nature can heal when given a chance. Wrong-food preparation, wrong food combining, poor mastication, over-eating, negative thinking and alkaline/acid balance in the body contribute to acidosis or toxicity, which then leads to sickness, disease and death. However, when we eat the proper food and maintain the proper PH in the body, our cells thrive nicely.

I decided to enjoy a long life by practicing daily, good, health habits. If I didn't feel well, I would re-group and see what natural laws were being broken and act accordingly. Food is the first important interest in life because upon it depend all other things. We should eat wholesome and natural foods and chew food to a liquid except for meats. A good policy is to quit eating while still hungry.

To achieve health, one must desire health with all of one's being. Desire alone will not restore your health but it will put one in the proper mind-frame to receive health. Affirm, everyday and in every way, I am getting better.

When we know and follow the principals of health, disease is then shut out. Disregarding the laws of health is unwise. Only those who do what is right are rewarded with the great gift of health. To end pain and sickness, we must earn health by daily, health habits. The potential for healing is in all of us; it is the negative influences that removes our health and shortens our lives. To experience lasting health, obey health laws and habits. The principle factor in healing is to plan to get well and then to stay well.

13

CHEMICAL EXPOSURE

Chemicals invade our environment on a daily basis by means of our homes, workplaces and other areas of life. Living in the modern age is great but it brings us into contact with thousands of chemicals; it is impossible to escape them. I found that when I was the sickest, they seemed to bother me the most. To this day, I cannot stand to walk down the detergent aisles at the department stores.

When I became well, I walked through the house, room to room, and took inventory. I immediately knew that things needed to change. Chemical products were everywhere in the form of dyes, solvents, curtains, carpets, furniture, cleaning supplies and more. Realizing that it would be impossible to eliminate all chemicals, I opted to get rid of as many as humanly possible. I figured that this wouldn't hurt my seasonal allergies. Inside the home were chemicals to clean floors, sinks, tubs, tile, toilets, glass, carpets, furniture, dishes stove, laundry, the air, etc. I cleaned out all products from under the sinks and in the closets. Some chemical products were eliminated all together while most were moved to the garage, out of the living quarters. I threw out harmful products in lieu of more natural ones. Many, safer products were already in the cabinets such as, baking soda, salt, vinegar and oils. I searched catalogs, the Internet and the health stores for safe, cleaning supplies. Whenever chemicals were utilized, I minimized exposure time, wore protective clothing/masks, gloves and used ventilation.

The following is the warning on the back of one, simple, window cleaner, Warning; can cause severe eye irritation, may cause respiratory tract irritation and in extreme case mild central nervous system depression characterized by flushing, headache, dizziness or nausea. Repeated exposure can have cumulative effects. Also, on the back were first aid instructions for the eyes, skin, if inhaled or if ingested. It stated to call the local poison control center in case of emergencies. It also included an 800 number in case the family pet happened to get poisoned. Wow, a person would have to be nuts to use this product in the home. The really bad products have these warnings while other products only list the ingredients knowing that most people will not bother to find out what the ingredients mean. What we don't know may be just as dangerous as what we do know.

After the household products were under control, next came the personal items. These products too were inventoried in amazement. The morning ritual for most consists of toothpaste mouthwash, soap, body wash, shampoo, conditioner, hair tonics, sprays, shaving cream, facial products, lotions, make-up, perfume, deodorant, powder and the occasional, hair color, with not a though going into what is in these products. For the most part, this process is repeated in the evening.

Whenever possible, less chemical products should be used, especially on the body. My recommendation is to start reading label and learn about the ingredients and the effect they have on the body. As a general rule, if you can't pronounce it, why would you want to place it in or on the body? Most health stores and some department stores have wonderful, cleaning products such as castile soap, shampoos, conditioners, hair color, and lotion, fluoride-free toothpaste and much more. Even the dollar stores have wonderful products for health such as, loofa, sea salt, baking salt, oatmeal, vinegar, soaps, spices, Epsom salt. etc. One can use baby products, which have fewer chemicals and are gentler to the body.

14

ELIMINATION OF HEAVY METALS

Metals can cause great harm to the human body and many people may be unaware of common products that they are in. Daily, we are exposed to aluminum, fluoride, cadmium and mercury. Some of the most common sources of aluminum are deodorants, antacids, baking powder, food additives, aluminum cookware, foil, drinking water and aluminum Christmas trees and other decorative items.

Aluminum has been implicated with Alzheimer's disease, Parkinson's disease, soft bones, anemia, dementia and nervous system disorders. Aluminum expose is one of the easiest to eliminate by not using the products, which contain aluminum.

Another element that most of us are exposed too on a daily basis is fluoride. Have Americans been given a bum steer in regard to fluoride? In my research, I found that fluoride has a long history dating back to 1886. It is the by-product of various manufacturing processes. In the 1930 in Belgium, many were killed due to an airborne release of fluoride at a factory and in America, we too have experienced fluoride casualties. In the 1940's it was properly classified as a poison but it was needed for the war effort to produce nuclear weapons. Today fluoride in found in water, sodas, fruit drinks, soups, and many strong cleaning supplies and in Prozac, which is called Fluoxetine.

Starting in the 1940's, fluoride was introduced into the American water supply. The question to ask is how did fluoride, a known poison, mutate into a harmless element and turn up in our water supply? An ex-fluoride employee ended up in Washington and was powerful enough to get this idea implemented. Next, to make matters worse, in the 1950's fluoride was added to toothpaste and it has been there ever since. This being a slick move to dispose of a hazardous waste, now the unsuspecting American public is paying for fluoride in more ways than one. The Food and Drug Administration (FDA) has never approved the use of fluoride by humans. Numerous countries from around the world have banned the use of fluoride in their drinking water.

Studies have shown that fluoride does not prevent cavities and can cause fluorosis, a toxic fluroine poisoning with white and spotty teeth. Approximately only one-half of all fluoride that enters the body can be eliminated, the rest remains to deplete the calcium reserves of the body, which leads to weak bones and fractures. Statistics also reveal that fluoridated communities have higher cancer rates than non-fluoridated ones.

Fluoride is an active ingredient in many pesticides. Each year there are thousands of calls to the poison control centers related to the ingestion of fluoride. Shockingly, there is enough fluoride in one tube of toothpaste to kill a child under nine years of age. Have you ever noticed what is on the back of fluoride toothpaste; Warning keep out of reach of children under six years of age. If more than used for brushing is accidentally swallowed, get medical help or contact a poison control center right away. Active ingredient sodium fluoride 0.24%. In the directions it says do not swallow!!! It sounds as though this fluoride was properly classified as a toxin to begin with. At normal, shopping centers, it is impossible to find fluoride-free toothpaste. Baking soda is a natural alternative or fluoride-free toothpaste may be purchased at the health stores.

Lastly, the American Dental Association has not quite been up to par in regards to the effects of mercury in amalgams. Mercury is the second, most toxic element on the planet, yet why do we walk around with it in our mouths? Amalgam fillings, which contain mercury, have been shown to emit it 50 years after being extracted from the mouth. Every time one chews, grins or eats this mercury can be released into the bloodstream. It then ends up in the brain, pituitary and other organs. Pregnant women with amalgam fillings have the potential to transfer this mercury to the fetus.

Years ago, while working in the dental field, I had to be routinely blood tested for mercury because we mixed the dental fillings with it. I don't see how anyone could deny that mercury is a health hazard.

Mercury has been associated with all of the following health problems:

memory loss
Alzheimer's
autism
nervousness
headaches

kidney damage
muscle problems
diarrhea
vomiting
mood disorder
increased heart rate
increased blood pressure
breathing problems
hallucinations
birth defects
bleeding gums
loose teeth
copper taste

Some of the most common sources of mercury are amalgam fillings, being the number one source, vaccinations, certain seafood, cosmetics, powder, antiseptics, chemicals and mercury thermometers. To prevent mercury poisoning, do not have mercury fillings, eat fish from a fish farm and eat seafood that has fins.

Oral chelation or IV treatment chelation therapy can assist with metal removal. Some dentists are specially trained in the removal of amalgam fillings. The International Academy of Oral Medicine and Toxicology, IOAMT, lists dentists who are trained to effectively remove these old-style fillings and replace them with a modern composite.

According to Dr. Hal Huggins, the immune system should be reinforced with antioxidants, vitamins, minerals and dietary changes before and after the procedure. This helps not to flood the system with released mercury during the procedure. Dr. Mercola's website recommends that before the fillings are removed, a detoxification protocol be given with the addition of helpful bacteria, chlorrella, garlic, MSM, cilantrol, minerals and diet, hychrochloric acid and antioxidants.

Some natural means to rid the body of mercury is to take NAC, glutathione and glutamic acid. Nevertheless, as long as mercury filling remains in the teeth, one will never be free of the effects of mercury.

15

EFFECT OF ELECTROMAGNETIC FIELDS

Electromagnetic fields (EMF) are electric and magnetic fields, which are generated in the vicinity of power lines, mobile phones, towers and other electrical equipment. EMF's refer to the 60 hertz fields associated with alternating current. In the 1990's, the EPA stated that EMF should be classified as a probable, human carcinogen. Studied have linked leukemia, lymphoma and cancer of the nervous system to EMF's.

Dr. David Carpenter believes that 30% of all childhood cancers are related to EMF's. Children are more susceptible to the effects of these fields because their cells are still growing and dividing. Humans are exposed to these fields on a daily basis at home, work and any other location where electrical power is generated. Common sources of EMF's are televisions, computers, electric razors, hairdryers, microwaves, fluorescent lights, telephones, electric blankets, clocks, etc. It is impossible for us to escape these fields but we must realize that they exist and be aware of the potential danger that they present to our health.

A way to determine one's exposure to these invisible fields is to purchase a gauss meter, which measures EMF's. A gauss meter measures in units called milligauss (mg). Obviously the closer one is to the source, the higher the reading will be. A meter may be used to determine "hot spots" in the home and these items may be relocated or eliminated if possible. To reduce exposure to EMF's, stay way from appliances when in use, reduce the time spent in their fields and avoid high sources such as electric appliances and blankets.

The Tools for Wellness website offers personal devices to wear to protect from EMF's and also a unit called a "Safe Space", which is designed to clear and balance the environment by addressing EMF, geopathic and other imbalanced energies in the environment. It works by changing the polarity of EMF from negative to positive and it resonates with the frequency patterns associated with a normal, healthy body. Equipment is available to measure milligauss of appliances and for those concerned about the safety of cellular phones, diodes are available to place on the phone to assist with this matter.

16

BIO-OXIDATIVE AND OZONE THERAPIES

Bio-oxidative therapies are therapies, which may be administered via an IV or by the ingesting pills. These treatments can help to oxidize toxins, kill bacteria, viruses and help to improve the immune system. Chelation Therapy has its origins way back in 1893 and a French chemist won the Nobel Prize in 1913 for his theory of chelates.

In 1935 the Germans produced ethyl-diamine-diamine-tetra-acetate, EDTA. It was found that EDTA removed poisonous gas compounds in humans. The navy has used it to treat sailors exposed to lead poisoning. In the 1960's EDTA was stockpiled in the United States for wartime usage. According to "The Lancet", hydrogen peroxide IV treatments were successfully used following World War I to treat a pneumonia epidemic. In the 1940's, Father Richard Wilhelm promoted these treatments and founded the "Educational Concern for Hydrogen Peroxide", ECHO. Dr. Charles Farr, Nobel Prize winner in medicine, has shown that hydrogen peroxide stimulates enzymes throughout the body, causing the arteries to dilate and increases the flow of blood.

Today, hydrogen peroxide and other chelates are given to patients mainly via an IV solution. Well over 50 years, Nobel Prize winner in medicine, Dr. Otto Warburg, demonstrated that the basic difference between the normal cell and the cancer cell was that both need energy from glucose but the normal cell requires oxygen while the cancer cell does not. This finding is one of the reasons for chelation therapy, to supply the body with additional oxygen thus allowing the body to ward off infections and cancers. I found chelation therapy to be a most beneficial treatment.

One must remember that hydrogen peroxide is not foreign to our bodies, in fact, our bodies produce it. These treatments are not a magical, cure-for-all but with other significant life-style changes, they certainly can help. The International Bio-oxidative Medicine Foundation (IBOM) is headed by Dr. Charles Farr and one may call 817 481-9772 for information about locating a physician trained in these procedures. An excellent book about this therapy is Forty Something For Ever by Harold Brecher and Arline Brecher.

Ozone (O3) is a natural and colorless gas, which gives that fresh smell after a rainstorm. Ozone oxidizes molds, pathogens, bacteria, viruses, etc. Ozone is a wonderful sterilizing agent, which is five times more effective than chlorine. Over 2,000 cities of the world use ozone to purify their drinking water. Medically, ozone is used in Germany, Russia, Cuba, Mexico and other countries around the world to treat viruses and bacterial infections.

Over 100 years ago, Nikola Tesla invented and patented a cold-plasma ozone generator. Today these machines are available on the Internet. I own Dr. Katz's AktivOxigen Ozonator, which is designed to ozonate liquids and oils. Ozonated water can be used to clean items such as toothbrushes, hairbrushes and other items. Ozonated water can be used to clean counters, sinks, laundry, and other areas of the home. It is an excellent wash for fresh fruits and vegetables and ozonated water is a natural, refreshing drink. Ozonated oil takes longer to produce but it will last for years. This oil makes a good ointment for skin problems such as cuts, bites, rashes etc. Ozone has been used to treat wounds, nerve gas, to purify blood, and much more. According to Dr. Katz, as far back as 1929, at least 114 diseases were treated with ozone and today, 16 nations used it. Ozone is extremely safe and effective when used properly.

17

THE BENEFITS OF EXERCISE

Eat right and exercise
Dr. Lenoard McCoy
Star Trek

Proper exercise stands out as a prominent factor in good health. Metabolic changes, which take place in the body create wastes or ash, which must be removed to prevent the clogging up of the machinery caused by toxins. If these toxins are not removed, life cannot be prolonged. The only successful eliminative process is by nature's way, which is by activity. Most of us get plenty of exercise for our arms and legs in our daily activity. However, most of us fail to give our trunk and interior muscles exercise, which results in premature death.

When we know why we grow old, we then have the necessary knowledge to stay young. Our bodies, being composed of millions of cells, come into being through the air we take in, the liquids we drink and the foods that we eat; by the process of digestion and assimilation, these elements are then converted into cellular tissue. Our cells live briefly, fulfill their mission and then die leaving dead matter that must be eliminated. The chief purpose of exercise is to assist in the removal of this waste material. Exercise also aids in forcing through the lymph system to the blood, suitable material to be supplied to every part of the body. Exercise is the chief means of eliminating toxins and thus gives the germicidal properties of the blood a chance to work.

REBOUNDING

All of us have of have seen trampolines in store and backyards all over America but have you ever stopped to consider the health benefits that can be derived from jumping up and down on them? Rebounding, jumping up and down on a trampoline, is not new, in fact, in the 1920's it was known that the trampoline contributed to the organization of visual perception better than any other known device.

Approximately, 36% of the fluids of the body is lymph. The purpose of the lymph is to remove wastes and bring nutrients to the cells. Rebounding is an excellent way to circulate the lymph through the body, especially since the lymph doesn't have any vessels to do so. Rebounding changes the "G" force or pressure of the body. During the jump, the bounce causes the lymph to flow and the bottom of the bounce squeezes the toxins out so that the body can be cleansed.

Some of the health benefits of rebounding are, its low trauma to the body, circulation of oxygen, toning the internal organs, improving cardiovascular health, and helping the endocrine, metabolic and the immune systems. The National Aeronautics and Space Administration (NASA) has incorporated rebounding in its program.

There are several types of rebounders. Some are portable and fold up for easy transport. Some have a balance bar and many offer a book and video of exercises. Rebounding is fun, doesn't require a great deal of time, effort, or special equipment or clothing to reap the health benefits. The best thing is that one can do something positive for one's health while watching the television or listening to music, all in the comfort of home. I try to use my rebounder for a few minutes each day.

For further information about rebounding, contact the American Institute of Reboundology at 1-888-464-5867(jump). An excellent book about rebounding is The Miracles of Rebound Exercise by Albert E. Carter, a pioneer in the field of rebounding.

CHI MACHINES

Chi machines are "swing" machines, which work by swinging the legs back in forth in a lateral position, similar to how a fish swims. The procedure is easy one lay on one's back and places the ankles onto the machine. The chi machine gently swings the body side to side removing toxins, oxygenating the spine while improving digestion. This machine can help to increase metabolism and the immune system.

Using a chi machine for 15 minutes is equivalent to walking for one and one-half hours in terms of oxygenation to the body. I use the Chi Vitalizer and have it to be a great aid to my exercise program. This exercise is great for those who don't have a lot of time to devote but want to get some exercise in. This machine has various speeds that one can work up too and it also comes with a timer.

WALKING

Open-air exercise or good, old-fashioned walking is one of the best and safest exercises that one can do. It reminds me of an old Chubby Checker song, Twenty Miles; he walked 20 miles every day to see his girl. How many miles would we walk for anything?

Walking is good exercise because it calls into the contractile powers of the heart and arteries; while calling the muscles into action, the quicker one walks the better. Exercising in the open air can help to cheer one up and take one's mind of one's troubles while enjoying the sights along the way.

The only required is a good pair of walking shoes and to be comfortable dresses. However, exercising should not be undertaken immediately after a meal.

18

HEALTHY SKIN

While researching health issues, I discovered that the skin is the body's largest eliminative organ, consisting of three layers and has over seven million pores. It is impossible to prick the skin without producing pain and causing a flow of blood within. One purpose of our skin is to regulate the temperature of the body. Two-thirds of the food and drink taken into the system is eliminated through the medium of the skin, while the bowels, lungs and kidneys pass off the remaining one-third.

When perspiration is arrested for a day or two, the blood will be charged with impurities to an almost incredible amount and disease will result due to waste matter not being removed. Cold applied to the skin or continued exposure to a cold atmosphere or decreased perspiration produces a bowel complaint, inflammation in the chest or some other internal organ. When the skin fails to function properly, the whole body suffers because noxious waste is left in the blood, causing a great weight to be placed on one's health.

Medical personnel place great weight upon the bowel movements, however, the skin secretes one to two pounds per day of waste matter and is an important organ. Therefore, there is a great necessity for keeping the pores of the skin clean. One should bathe first thing in the morning, scrubbing the skin and the bottom of the feet well with a loofa or a brush, followed by drying with a vigorous rub with a coarse towel. This will strengthen the nervous system, remove perspired matter, which has been passed off while sleeping; if not remove, it will be reabsorbed and recharges the blood with poisonous matter.

I dry brush my skin with a natural brush to increase the temperature of the skin and help to assist with toxin removal. The soaking of the feet is an important way to expel toxins from the body. I use footbaths and they can be used to help draw colds out of the body. The water should be as hot as can be stood and soak the feet 10 to 15 minutes. A tablespoon of dry mustard powder can be added to assist with this.

Another way to rid the body of toxins is by the use of "de-tox" pads on the soles of the feet. These pads contain natural ingredients, which assist with drawing out toxins. They are placed on the bottom of the feet before retiring at night and in the morning, one will be amazed at the toxins on these pads in the morning.

Years ago, I discovered that many health benefits can be derived from the use of infrared heat. This heat or energy can penetrate up to three inches in the body and some of its health benefits are, raising temperatures in tissues, expanding capillary vessels, rejuvenating cells, removing toxins reducing pain, helping the lymphatic and immune system. Infrared light is natural, safe and does not burn like ultraviolet light does.

Many types of equipment are available from hand-held units, mats, lamps and saunas. The Far Infrared Mineral Lamp (FIM) or also called the TDP lamp was introduced in the 1980's for clinical use. It is sometimes called the "miracle lamp" because it has assisted millions of people around the world with pain issues. The TDP lamp is a FDA approved medical device and is acceptable for insurance billing. However, the best news is that it is available without a prescription and may be ordered on the Internet.

The TDP or "miracle lamp" is not a normal lamp but rather a black, ceramic plate, which is impregnated with 33 elements, essential to the human body. When heated, the mineral plate emits a band of infrared light, which is easily absorbed by the body. There are several models of this lamp to range from desktop models to those on wheels for easy transport. The operation of the unit is simple and a timer is included.

An excellent book about the mineral lamp is Pain Free with Infrared Mineral Therapy by Kara Lee Schoonover. Since minerals are critical to one's health, this is an excellent and safe way to incorporate them into one's health regime.

Another great product is the infrared sauna, which offers all the above health benefits. Home units are now designed to snap together and they work quite well. They may be purchased with ionizers, aromatherapy, and stereos.

I frequently use the "miracle lamp" when I have isolated areas of pain. We were able to purchase an infrared sauna and have incorporated it into our exercise program. We were lucky enough to have some extra space downstairs and converted a room into an exercise room, which houses our machines, weights and the sauna.

19

ENERGY MEDICINE

Energy medicine or Bioelectric medicine has its roots back to D'Arsnonval and Tesla. However, D'Arsonal and Oudin discovered the physical effects of these currents. Nagelschmidt of Berlin was the first to announce a technique of therapeutic treatments. Royal Rife from America was curing cancer with his equipment until he was jailed for doing so.

Long ago, it was stated what a glorious achievement it would be to find a way of producing fever and controlling it as a remedial agent in the treatment of chronic diseases. Through the efforts of the above men, temperatures were raised and controlled to parts of the body. Hippocrates, The Father of Medicine, proclaimed, give me fever and I can cure anything. Hyperemia is called into play by nature more often than any reparative process. There is no gland of the body that cannot be reached and its function profoundly influenced by electric energy.

Electricity and other physical measures are potent agents for good in the treatment of disease and it is safe and sound. From an electrophysiological standpoint, the body is the most delicate and wonderful apparatus that we know. The body has generators, rheostats, condensers, transformers and more. It produces amperes, coulombs and watts. The skin presents a resistance of thousands of ohms. The body is full of cells, which develop alternating, sinuosidal, static, inductive and oscillary currents. Its diatherimic apparatus converts mechanical energy into heat. The body as a whole exhibits a polarity, which is positive but may be changed to negative by surrounding objects, etc. It receives electrical charges and dispersed them. It has electrical currents open and closed. While body currents may flow through almost any tissue, the nerves are the all-important conductors.

When a normal tissue takes on pathological change, it becomes an insulator of body current. The body currents, being the main factor in nutrition, it is logical that tissues deprived of these currents will take on degeneration. In fatigue of animals or vegetable matter, the polarity of the currents are reversed. A high-frequency current induces hyperemia and changes take place, which increase nutrition, as long as toxic influences are not brought within the cells.

Toxic agents can be overcome and thus prevents the cells from becoming doomed. After years of Electro-physiology research, it was determined that:

1. Everything living, whether animal or vegetable has a well-defined electrical system.

2. The edible part of a fruit or vegetable is the positive element, which yields a positive galvanometric reaction.

3. Every plant, fruit, vegetable, tuber and seed is an electrical cell and cannot be polarized or discharged so long as it remains structurally perfect.

4. The skin, peel, rind or jacket of fruits and vegetables is the nature of an insulting substance primarily designed for the conservation of their electrical energy.

When the entire bloodstream is thoroughly heated, there is a rise in temperature, acceleration of pulse rate, increased volatile waste and elimination of carbon dioxide. As an equalizer of the circulation, electrical current has no peer. The vitality of all tissues from almost any cause is eliminated.

In 1934, George Lakhovsky with the aid of Nekola Tesla built a multiple wave oscillator (MWO). This machine was used to treat numerous diseases. The MWO works on the principle of harmonic frequencies within the human body to bring about as normal state. This machine is still marketed today on the Internet.

Dr. Robert Beck, a physicist, specialized in the making of energy devices. In the 1970's and 1980's, he developed a device called the Brain Tuner to heal and stimulate neuro-transmitters. Next, he worked on the lymph system by developing a magnetic pulser and a blood electrification/purifier device.

He worked with HIV and AIDS patients. His protocol is referred to as the "Beck Protocol." Bob Beck's original machine or black box electrified the blood by placing two electrodes on the skin over arteries in the ankles or the wrist with leads or wires running to the box. The treatment was for one to two hours per day for five to eight weeks. Viruses, bacteria, fungus and parasites in the blood were neutralized or killed. This machine became the Blood Electrifier Machine.

Later, he found that after a year, some of the test subjects became re-infected. He concluded that some of the viruses were hiding in the lymph fluid and had made their way back into the bloodstream. To solve this problem, he invented the Magnetic Pulser, which creates a momentary current, causing a contraction of the lymph vessels and forces lymph movement, thus pushing the germs into the bloodstream to be zapped. The combination of both machines resulted in the elimination of viruses. The Magnetic Pulser by Sota Instruments is made per Dr. Beck's design. The above units are safe to use and use less current than the current approved TENS units.

Some companies sell individual units or a combination of the Bob Beck Pulser/Blood Electrifier and a Hulda Clark Zapper such as, the RSG-1 Combo Research Signal Generator. For those not familiar with this technology, I would recommend that one go to Forbidden Cures on line, which has a wealth of information.

In 1990 at the Albert Einstein College of Medicine, Dr. Kaali and Dr. Lyman discovered that after exposure to an electrical current, HIV suppressed its capability to induce the formation of syncytica. In other words, HIV was reduced by 90%. Doctors Kaali and Lyman received a patent for this discovery, #518873, which states, "provide electric current flow through the blood sufficient to render the bacteria, virus, parasites and/or fungus ineffective to infect or affect normal, healthy cells while maintaining the biological usefulness of the blood or others fluids."

Bioelectric energy has been successfully used in this country around the late 1880's and up into the 1930's, until pharmaceuticals became more popular. The FDA has approved the use of electrical devices for what is termed "personal research." There are many types and makers of these machines on the Internet. Many websites offers instructions about its use and its long history.

20

BREAST HEALTH

Years ago, I stopped getting annual mammograms due to the radiation exposure, pain issues and because there are other tests available, which can detect changes in the breast tissue years before a mammogram.

Every year most women are urged to undergo mammography for breast, cancer prevention. However, when it comes to radiation exposure, there is no safe level. The Department of Health and Human Services in "The Report on Carcinogens" lists x-rays and gamma radiation as "known human carcinogens." Breast cancer detection is critical but at what expense? Each year over 180,000 women are diagnosed and 44,000 women die from breast cancer. This is the leading cause of death in the 44-45 age group. A Canadian study revealed that mammograms did not have any positive effect on the mortality rate of women in this age group.

Compared to other cancers, breast cancer is a slow, growing cancer and may take years to develop. Giving younger women yearly mammograms increases their cumulative radiation exposure and risks of developing cancer. In some premenopasal women, there is an oncogene, which makes them even more sensitive to radiation. "The Lancet" reported that since the introduction of mammograms, ductal carcinoma in situ has substantially increased.

In the book "Politics of Cancer", Dr. Samuel S. Epstein states that the risk of cancer increases per x-ray. This is very alarming since yearly mammograms can consist of four to 16 exposures depending upon such factors as the density and shape of the breast. Based on only four x-rays, each breast is exposed to an average of 250mr (millirem), a measurement of ionizing radiation, times two exposures per breast equates to 1,000mr or one rad (radiation absorbed dose). To place all of this into its proper prospective, the average human receives approximately 100mr to the **whole** body from naturally occurring, background radiation each year. In other works, the damage to the body is much less due to the lower exposure rate and because the radiation is spread out over the entire body and not to one body part.

Besides the cumulative, radiation risks, some of the drawbacks to mammograms are pain, compression of a potential tumor and the false positives, which arise and lead to unnecessary stress and biopsies. How might one avoid all this? There are many ways to prevent breast cancer such as, good eating habits, taking supplements, eliminating toxins, limiting exposure to estrogen, self/clinical examinations and noninvasive procedures such as, ultra sound and thermography.

The Father of Medicine, Hippocrates, stated in 400BC, "In whatever part of the body that heat or cold is felt, the disease is there to be discovered." Decades ago it was found that when a tumor was over the breast, it would measure warmer than healthy tissues; due to the tumor producing its own blood supply to feed upon. This is where thermography can be beneficial. Thermography works on the principle of heat using high-definition, infrared technology. Thermography detects physiological changes that take place in the breast tissue, which has been shown to correlate with the presence of cancer or a precancerous state.

In 1982 the FDA approved thermography for breast, cancer screening. The procedure is simple and is performed in the physician's office. The patient disrobes from the waist up and is conditioned to the surrounding, room temperature for 15 minutes. Next, the patient's hands are submerged into cold water for one minute and the first, set of images are taken. This is not a normal photograph but rather is color images, which shows an outline that the trained professional may interpret.

Dr. Alan D. Lieberman from the Center of Occupational and Environmental Medicine stated, "Thermography can detect physiological changes in the breast tissue and changes up to 10 years before a tumor develops and can be detected by a mammogram thus allowing for early intervention." He went on to say, "The procedure is painless, effective and is safe for younger and pregnant women."

Why should women continue to be exposed to years and years of needless radiation exposure when other, FDA approved, screening techniques are available and effective?

21

A WONDER DRUG

Drugs serve a useful purpose but I do not take them unless absolutely necessary. However, that being said, I would like to introduce you to a truly, wonderful drug, which is helping so many people with many immune deficiency diseases. Low Dose Naltrexone (LDN) has been around over 20 years and may prove to a drug of choice for the future.

Although, LDN, is a FDA approved drug, many physicians are unaware of its great benefits to those who suffer from immune deficiency diseases. Originally Naltrexone was given in 50mg doses to treat heroin or opium addicts. Lately, it has been in the news for helping with alcohol addiction. It works by blocking the endorphin levels that are produced by the brain and the adrenaline glands. It had been known that the brain contains receptors for chemicals produced by the poppy plant. In the 1970's, while researching drug addition, scientists discovered that the brain produced neurochemicals, which are more potent than morphine, opium, and heroin and share the same receptors with these drugs. These naturally, produced brain chemicals are called endorphins, which the body releases in times of stress and to induce mood elevations. There are some natural means to stimulated the release of endorphins by strenuous running, cycling, swimming and eating foods, which contain the amino acid L-Phenylalamine such as, almonds, bananas, cheese, lima beans, peanuts, pumpkin or sesame seeds.

Every cell of the immune system has receptors for these agents. It was discovered that people who suffer from immune disorders such as, cancer, AIDS, chronic fatigue, Lou Gehrig's Disease, fibromylagia, lupus, multiple sclerosis, etc. have low endorphin levels, which causes poor immune function. When the immune system is low, the body forgets to attack the bacteria, fungus, viruses and cancer cells. When this happens, the body may also begin to attack itself. LDN restores the endorphin levels to normal so that the immune system can do the job that it was designed to do. LDN boosts the immune system by elevating the endorphin levels thus helping to fight off diseases. This is done without side effects, drug resistance, it's non-additive, it works, is inexpensive and easy to take. Optimum immune results are seen after several months of use.

Dr. Bernard Bihari from New York City discovered in 1985 that lower doses of LDN, 3mg, enhanced the body's T-cells. He later determined that 4.5mg was a more effective dose. In studies with rats and humans, cancer cells have has been inhabited by using endorphins and LDN. It is believed that the increased levels of endorphin induced by LDN causes the death of the cancer cell. In 2004 Dr. Bihari had treated over 400, multiple sclerosis patients with LDN. Of the total, only two patients showed new disease while on LDN. Great success has also been found in stopping certain cancers in their tracks. In the 1990's LDN was studied for autism and positive results were found in the areas of mood, cognition, language and social skills.

A "compounding pharmacy" should fill LDN, one in which the medicines are especially prepared by pharmacists to meet the patient's, individual needs. Since most of the endorphins are produced at night between two a.m. and four a.m., the medicine is taken at night between nine p.m. to midnight; thus tripling the endorphin levels in the body and all of the next day the levels are restored to normal. A great place to have the LDN filled is at Skip's Pharmacy in Florida and they have a website, which makes ordering easy. They provide excellent service for this need.

For further information about LDN, go to lowdosenaltrexone.org. This drug has been a lifesaver for me.

22

THE MIND CONNECTION

**All the literature of medicine, whether of ancient or modern times,
Abounds in illustration of the power of the mind over body in health and in
disease.**
Warren Hilton

This very important chapter was reserved for last because no amount of detoxification, restoration, or maintenance will be effective without the proper, mental attitude towards health. To paraphrase Abraham Lincoln, man is about as happy as he makes up his mind to be and to add to that, one is about as healthy as one makes up one's mind to be.

To elaborate on this point, let's cover some very real issues in regards to the mind and health. William Shakespeare wisely stated, "There is nothing good or bad that thinking makes it so." Science has long known about the placebo effect, which is Latin for "I shall please." "Webster's Dictionary" defines placebo as, a substance having no pharmacological effect but given merely to satisfy a patient who supposes it to be medicine. In essence, it is a fake medicine. Nevertheless, this did not stop the medicine man of yesteryear from peddling their sugar and alcoholic tonics. Simply stated, placebos are mental crutches. There aren't any curative ingredients in them. It is the belief by the recipient that it will work, which causes it to work. Time and time again this has been proven in controlled, medical studies. The placebo can work like the real McCoy; it is the belief of the patient, which heals.

Personally, I have had experience with this effect. One occasion I had reactions to vaccinations, which required medication. Later in the same year, I was given more vaccinations and had another reaction, more medications and this time great pain lasting for months. During this time, I was enrolled in a study of "electrolyzed water" for the Wellness Directory of Minnesota. Since I had litmus paper, I decided to play detective and test the PH of all the water in the house. I measured the PH of the study water, the kitchen tap water and the bottled water, which is what we normally drank. In comparing all of the samples, the study's water was very high, off the chart. Naturally, I concluded that I was drinking the real stuff and not the placebo.

For eight days, I religiously guzzled down this water and experienced remarkable results, starting from day one. All eight days I remained pain free and did not get the flu bug that 11 of my friends and family unfortunately suffered through. I was on the "wonder" product and couldn't possibly get sick! As luck would have it, I was on the placebo, tap water from Minnesota, which naturally had a very high PH. Cognizant of the truth, my belief system had been shattered and to add insult to injury, my pain returned. My husband was quite amused by all of this. In fact, he wanted to bottle and to sell this Minnesota water as he stated that we were paying $60/month for water that the PH wasn't any better. After getting over my initial disappointment, I too had to see the humor in all of this. This whole incident reaffirmed my belief in the concept of mind over matter and that the most important aspect of one's health is one's mental attitude.

Armed with the revelation of the above test, I decided to try to mentally work through my pain issues. In reality, if tap water from Minnesota could relieve pain, then by the same token actively concentrating on being pain free should not be an impossible feat.

Another real effect to health is something called the nocebo effect. Robert Collier stated, "When something seems wrong with the functioning of your body, the place to investigated is your subconscious mind." The first cousin of the placebo is the nocebo. This term came into vogue in the 1990's. "Webster's New World Medical Dictionary" defines nocebo as, a negative placebo effect, when patients taking medications experience adverse side effects unrelated to the specific pharmacological action of the drug. The nocebo effect is associated with the person's prior expectations of adverse effects from treatments as well as with in which the person learns from prior experience to associate a medication with certain somatic symptoms. Nocebo stems from the Latin for "I shall harm." Robert S. and Michele R. Root Berstein stated "Research has also shown that the nocebo effect can reverse the body's response to true medical treatment from positive to negative."

Brian Reid noted in the "Special to the Washington Post", 30 April 2002, that researchers discovered that, "Women who believed that they were prone to heart disease were nearly four times as likely to die as women with similar risk factors who didn't hold such fatalistic views. The higher risk of death, in other words, had nothing to do with the usual health disease culprits-age, blood pressure, cholesterol, weight. Instead it tracked closely with belief; think sick be sick." The nocebo effect has been documented in numerous studies. The white coat syndrome could fall under this category. How many people get anxious by just going to the doctor or the dentist? The mental anxiety of sticks, probes, etc. can cause alarm to even the seasoned among us. My brother-in-law is a classic example. He has passed out from having his blood pressure checked. The procedure in itself is harmless but the mental aspect is worse than the event. Job proclaimed that which I have feared has come upon me and the great Psalmist stated, as a man thinketh in his heart so is he.

Another classification to mull over is hypochondria. "Webster's Dictionary" defines hypochondria as an abnormal condition characterized by a depressed emotional state and imaginary ill health, referable to the physical condition of the body or one of its parts. Hypochondriac is a person who worries or talks excessively about his health. My mother-in-law, bless her heart, is a first-class hypochondriac. Let anyone in the family complain of any ailment and she is immediately in competition with them. She has the problem, is getting the problem or she had it in the past. Her family physician now recognizes that this is a problem. We all laugh about it and try to choose our words more carefully or we will be opening up Pandora's Box.

Many harbor their aches and pains as old friends and love to introduce them to anyone who will listen. An old Chinese Proverb wisely says 5,000 will bet the flu but five times that will die from the fear of it. Theodore Roosevelt stated there is nothing to fear but fear itself.

Lastly, medconism, my terminology, is when one subscribes to the doctrine that medication is necessary to improve health or to sustain health. Oliver Wendell Holmes proclaimed, "That if 99 percent of all drugs we posses were thrown into the sea it would be a good thing for the human race, but rather hard on the fishes." Mind is the healer. Drugs can sometimes make it easier by removing obstruction and by killing off parasites.

Starting at a very young age and throughout our life, we are conditioned to take a pill for everything. Have a headache, take a pill, the back or leg hurts, take a pill, pill, and pill. When was the last time that you saw an advertisement for acid reflux, restless leg syndrome, over-active bladder, migraines, insomnia, constipation, hemorrhoids, diarrhea, toe fungus, erectile dysfunction and the list goes on and on. Isn't anything sacred? Today, thanks to the marvels of television, the well-informed patient can waltz into the doctor's office and tell the doctor what to prescribe. Makes one wonder why the doctor spent hours in class when he or she could have turned on the television to learn about drugs. Now days, the doctor can no longer give sound medical advise such as, lose weight, get some exercise, change your diet, take a vacation or the patient will be offended by not having been given a pill. In most cases the physician would do well to give a dummy pill so that the patient would get well sooner.

Our minds can receive commands from us and it has a wonderful ability to carry them out; every thought realizes itself subconsciously in the body. Wow, what a concept, we all have our own personal genie just waiting to grant us our wishes! Why not build on the idea of perfect health? The mind is capable of great healing. However, drugs can assist with this when needed. Most of us have not reached the ability to trust the body to heal its self. Many of us require our various crutches in life. Nevertheless, with or without them, first requires a belief in wellness.

Right thoughts, interests and self-confidence will keep you happy and healthy. If you think and believe in health, the subconscious mind will work for you to rebuild every cell of your anatomy. It is a law that the opinion that one holds of oneself will be reproduced outwardly in the body. Improper eating followed by improper thinking is the cause of sickness. Words expressed can actually attract the disease that one fears into one's life. No matter whether the mind is creating success or failure, it is creating. Remember your subconscious mind will move heaven and Earth to rebuild every cell of your anatomy so build on the idea of perfect health.

EPILOGUE

The preservation of health depends upon our daily, health habits. Days, weeks, months and years add up to either good or bad habits, which are reflected in our well being. Sickness is not natural but is produced mainly by violating the principles of health. Wrong diets, over-eating, lack of exercise, negative thinking and other negative influences destroy tissue and organs until sickness and premature death occurs.

Life is neutral, ever ready to give to us what we have the "vision" to demand. When we locate and correct our disease-producing habits, we become aligned to the principles of health. The potential is in all of us but we must strive to control our diets, negative thoughts, toxins and other bad influences to achieve our goal. When we change these negative influences, health will again be restored.

Another important issue to excellent health is one's mental attitude. When thoughts are negative in regard to health, one can actually attract disease into one's life. Remember, improper health habits along with improper thoughts are a sure combination to bring sickness into one's life.

Finally, there is no magic wand or easy pathway to health; it is a disciplined or dedicated climb, earned by our daily, health habits. By living according to natural law and by demanding the subconscious to rebuild every cell of our bodies, along the lines of perfect health, life will then give us what we have the faith to demand; then will we be healthy, happy and prosperous.

978-0-595-43152-6
0-595-43152-6

www.ingramcontent.com/pod-product-compliance
Lightning Source LLC
Chambersburg PA
CBHW030413290526
45785CB00004B/1988